AF764204

Adipose Tissue Homeostasis in Health and Disease

Edited by Féaron C. Cassidy

Published in London, United Kingdom

We are IntechOpen, the world's leading publisher of Open Access books

Built by scientists, for scientists

7,500+
Open access books available

196,000+
International authors and editors

215M+
Downloads

156
Countries delivered to

Our authors are among the
Top 1%
most cited scientists

12.2%
Contributors from top 500 universities

CLARIVATE ANALYTICS BOOK CITATION INDEX INDEXED

WEB OF SCIENCE™

Selection of our books indexed in the Book Citation Index in Web of Science™ Core Collection (BKCI)

Interested in publishing with us?
Contact book.department@intechopen.com

Numbers displayed above are based on latest data collected.
For more information visit www.intechopen.com

Adipose Tissue Homeostasis in Health and Disease
http://dx.doi.org/10.5772/intechopen.12358
Edited by Féaron C. Cassidy

Contributors
Alicia Mayeuf-Louchart, Amine Bouchekioua, Ana Soriano-Arroquia, Andrea Woodcock, Anna-Theresa Lipp, Anna Maria Ernst, Claudine Duggan, Dominik Tischer, Erwin Schimak, Féaron C. Cassidy, Hannelore Bauer, Hans-Christian Bauer, Marianne Steiner, Noor Bakour, Olivier Pourquié, Stephanie L. Annett

© The Editor(s) and the Author(s) 2025

The rights of the editor(s) and the author(s) have been asserted in accordance with the Copyright, Designs and Patents Act 1988. All rights to the book as a whole are reserved by INTECHOPEN LIMITED. The book as a whole (compilation) cannot be reproduced, distributed or used for commercial or non-commercial purposes without INTECHOPEN LIMITED's written permission. Enquiries concerning the use of the book should be directed to INTECHOPEN LIMITED rights and permissions department (permissions@intechopen.com).

Violations are liable to prosecution under the governing Copyright Law.

Individual chapters of this publication are distributed under the terms of the Creative Commons Attribution 3.0 License which permits commercial use, distribution and reproduction of the individual chapters, provided the original author(s) and source publication are appropriately acknowledged. If so indicated, certain images may not be included under the Creative Commons license. In such cases users will need to obtain permission from the license holder to reproduce the material. More details and guidelines concerning content reuse and adaptation can be found at http://www.intechopen.com/copyright-policy.html.

Notice

Statements and opinions expressed in the chapters are these of the individual contributors and not necessarily those of the editors or publisher. No responsibility is accepted for the accuracy of information contained in the published chapters. The publisher assumes no responsibility for any damage or injury to persons or property arising out of the use of any materials, instructions, methods or ideas contained in the book.

First published in London, United Kingdom, 2025 by IntechOpen
IntechOpen is the global imprint of INTECHOPEN LIMITED, registered in England and Wales, registration number: 11086078, 167-169 Great Portland Street, London, W1W 5PF, United Kingdom

For EU product safety concerns: IN TECH d.o.o., Prolaz Marije Krucifikse Kozulić 3, 51000 Rijeka, Croatia, info@intechopen.com or visit our website at intechopen.com.

British Library Cataloguing-in-Publication Data
A catalogue record for this book is available from the British Library

Adipose Tissue Homeostasis in Health and Disease
Edited by Féaron C. Cassidy
p. cm.
Print ISBN 978-1-83769-341-2
Online ISBN 978-1-83769-340-5
eBook (PDF) ISBN 978-1-83769-342-9

If disposing of this product, please recycle the paper responsibly.

Meet the editor

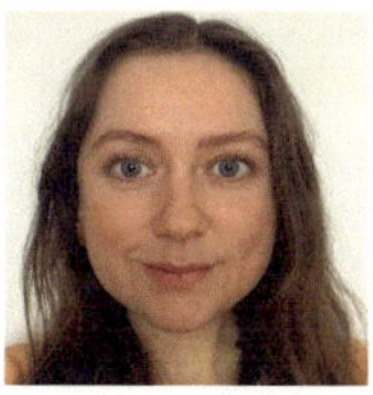

Dr. Féaron C. Cassidy currently works as a DOROTHY COFUND & Marie Skłodowska-Curie Fellow jointly between the Department of Medicine at Karolinska Institutet in Sweden and the Kathleen Lonsdale Institute for Human Health Research at Maynooth University in Ireland. Previously, Dr. Cassidy worked as a postdoctoral researcher at the Royal College of Surgeons Ireland (mRNA therapeutics for type 2 diabetes), at Maynooth University (obesity immunology) and at the National University of Ireland, Galway (mesenchymal stromal cells in type 2 diabetes). She completed her Ph.D. at the William Harvey Research Institute, Queen Mary University of London, on the topic of imprinted genes in adipose tissue development.

Contents

Preface

Adipose tissue has numerous, vital physiological functions, a topic discussed in the introductory chapter (Chapter 1). Its importance to health is evident from the impact observed when it is dysfunctional and the observation of evolutionary conservation of the gene signaling pathways that control its functions. For example, adipose tissue plays a role in disease risk from cancer to infection, as described here in Chapters 2 and 3, while SREBP and C/EBP have conserved functions from nematodes to mammals [1]. The varied functions of adipose tissue are split differentially between the different types of adipose tissue, which are categorized first by the predominant adipocyte type and then by deposition location. The first hierarchical split defines the two major types of adipose tissue - white adipose tissue and brown adipose tissue – based on a predominance of either white or brown adipocytes within the depot. These adipocyte types share common features but are developmentally distant. They are separated early in mesodermal differentiation, with brown adipocytes being more closely related to muscle than white adipocytes [2, 3]. Therefore, in this book the chapters have been grouped according to whether they discuss findings related to white or brown adipose tissue.

Despite the opposing roles of white and brown adipose tissue in fuel processing, it is also interesting to note the commonalities between them. All adipose tissue shares a set of highly specialized biochemical functions mediated by a shared set of genes which direct the synthesis and storage of triglycerides and the release of unesterified fatty acids – processes termed lipogenesis and lipolysis, respectively.

The most well-known function of adipose tissue is its capacity for lipid storage, a function performed by white adipocytes. This stored lipid acts as a fuel released by adipocytes according to energy demands, fluctuating throughout the day according to mealtimes and playing a crucial role in survival during longer periods of insufficient dietary intake. The adipocyte has evolved this specialized function of healthful lipid accumulation which alleviates the potentially harmful effects of aberrant lipid deposition in other tissues. Humans, with our extended energy-sequestering gestation and lactation periods, have a relatively large proportion of adipose tissue to body weight [4].

White adipose tissue is further classified according to its deposition at either subcutaneous or visceral levels and then further subclassified according to its anatomical location. These depots have shared and distinct functions, and their expansion and/or dysfunction lead to differential effects on metabolism and overall health. This can be observed by the differential effects on metabolic health of so-called apple- and pear-shaped obesity (whereby apple-shaped or central obesity is independently associated with metabolic ill health), as well as in lipodystrophies and lipedema (discussed in Chapter 4), which exhibit depot-specific onset and pathologies [5, 6]. The distinct phenotypes between these depots are dictated by both intrinsic factors (e.g. cellular developmental origin) and extrinsic factors (e.g. level of vasculature and nutrient exposure) [7, 8].

The brown color that eponymizes brown adipose tissue comes from the density of mitochondria and vascularization in this tissue [9]. This tissue releases heat in response to stimulation (e.g. via cold exposure or beta-adrenergic receptor) in a process independent from shivering and with its primary importance during infancy and hibernation [10–12]. This thermogenic capacity is a phenotype which can be acquired in white adipose when consistent stimulation of brown adipose thermogenesis is provided [13, 14]. While initially touted as a simple solution to the obesity crisis, therapeutic targeting of this pathway has proven not to be the anticipated silver bullet since stimulation of brown adipose tissue in humans results in minimal metabolic modification in conjunction with adverse effects [15, 16]. Further, chronic inflammation drives the browning of white adipose tissue in cachexia and is a contributor to death in those cases, emphasizing the caution required in targeting this pathway. The role of brown adipose tissue in metabolic health and the research unpicking the now-recognized complexity of targeting this pathway to improve health are discussed in Chapters 5 and 6.

The key role of adipose tissue in various diseases and disorders emphasizes the importance of understanding its biology. In order to develop therapeutics and disease biomarkers, it is essential to gain an understanding of the mechanisms of adipose tissue expansion and dysfunction. These topics are discussed by the expert authors in the chapters that follow.

Dr. Féaron C. Cassidy
Kathleen Lonsdale Institute for Human Health Research,
Department of Biology,
Maynooth University,
Co. Kildare, Ireland

Center for Infectious Medicine,
Department of Medicine,
Huddinge Karolinska Institute,
Huddinge, Sweden

References

[1] McKay RM, McKay JP, Avery L, Graff JM. C. elegans: A model for exploring the genetics of fat storage. Dev Cell. 2003;4(1)

[2] Wang C, Liu W, Nie Y, Qaher M, Horton HE, Yue F, et al. Loss of MyoD Promotes Fate Transdifferentiation of Myoblasts Into Brown Adipocytes. EBioMedicine. 2017;16

[3] Seale P, Bjork B, Yang W, Kajimura S, Chin S, Kuang S, et al. PRDM16 controls a brown fat/skeletal muscle switch. Nature. 2008;454(7207)

[4] Isler K. Adipose tissue in evolution. In: Adipose Tissue and Adipokines in Health and Disease: Second Edition. 2014

[5] Snijder MB, Dekker JM, Visser M, Bouter LM, Stehouwer CDA, Kostense PJ, et al. Associations of hip and thigh circumferences independent of waist circumference with the incidence of type 2 diabetes: The Hoorn Study. American Journal of Clinical Nutrition. 2003;77(5)

[6] Garg A. Lipodystrophies. Vol. 108, American Journal of Medicine. 2000

[7] Satoor SN, Puranik AS, Kumar S, Williams MD, Ghale M, Rahalkar A, et al. Location, location, location: Beneficial effects of autologous fat transplantation. Sci Rep. 2011;1

[8] Tran TT, Yamamoto Y, Gesta S, Kahn CR. Beneficial Effects of Subcutaneous Fat Transplantation on Metabolism. Cell Metab. 2008;7(5)

[9] Nnodim JO, Lever JD. Neural and vascular provisions of rat interscapular brown adipose tissue. American Journal of Anatomy. 1988;182(3)

[10] van Marken Lichtenbelt WD. Human Brown Adipose Tissue—A Decade Later. Obesity. 2021;29(7)

[11] Cannon B, Nedergaard J. Brown Adipose Tissue: Function and Physiological Significance. Vol. 84, Physiological Reviews. 2004

[12] Emorine LJ, Marullo S, Briend-Sutren MM, Patey G, Tate K, Delavier-Klutchko C, et al. Molecular characterization of the human β3-adrenergic receptor. Science (1979). 1989;245(4922)

[13] Lonçar D, Afzelius BA, Cannon B. Epididymal white adipose tissue after cold stress in rats I. Nonmitochondrial changes. Journal of Ultrastructure Research and Molecular Structure Research. 1988;101(2–3)

[14] Lončar D. Convertible adipose tissue in mice. Cell Tissue Res. 1991;266(1)

[15] Harb E, Kheder O, Poopalasingam G, Rashid R, Srinivasan A, Izzi-Engbeaya C. Brown adipose tissue and regulation of human body weight. Vol. 39, Diabetes/Metabolism Research and Reviews. 2023

[16] Munafò A, Frara S, Perico N, Di Mauro R, Cortinovis M, Burgaletto C, et al. In search of an ideal drug for safer treatment of obesity: The false promise of pseudoephedrine. Vol. 22, Reviews in Endocrine and Metabolic Disorders. 2021

Section 1

Introduction

Chapter 1

Introductory Chapter: On the Importance of Functional Adipose Tissue

Féaron C. Cassidy

1. Introduction

Obesity is an established global health concern due to the recognition and recording of the higher prevalence of predominantly metabolic pathologies in the population with obesity. Both rates of obesity and rates of those pathologies have been increasing in tandem globally for a number of decades, and are often but not exclusively coincident. Childhood obesity is the major predictor of adulthood obesity, and both predict risk of metabolic pathology on a population level. Prevention of obesity at any age has superior health outcomes and lower social and economic costs than obesity reversal. Targeted studies aimed at reversing obesity have identified a lack of long-term efficacy across interventional lifestyle modifications at a rate that would contraindicate their widespread uptake, while surgical and pharmaceutical interventions entail risk of adverse events, high financial burden, and low accessibility. Current preventative efforts to reduce the global burden of obesity-associated morbidity have focused on promoting healthy individual lifestyle choices and reformulation of processed foods to reduce sugar and fat content. Thus far these efforts have failed globally, and rates of obesity and metabolic disorders continue to increase. At the heart of our understanding of obesity as a health issue, is a loss of adipose tissue homeostasis associated with excess expansion and metabolic disruption. In order to progress our understanding of obesity and to improve public health, it is imperative to better understand adipose tissue physiology.

1.1 Functional adipose tissue is necessary for survival

Dysfunctional adipose tissue is associated with higher mortality – both in cases of excess and insufficiency. Epidemiolocally, the highest mortality by BMI is associated with being underweight [1]. In fact, it is not until a BMI of 36 (categorised as severe obesity) that increased mortality associated with excess weight is observed [1]. Evidence suggests that the overt focus on BMI and weight, including weight bias and stigma results in decreased screening and investigative testing, missed diagnoses, delayed treatment, and ultimately a contribution to morbidity and mortality in people with obesity that is independent of physiological risk [2–5]. Even within cardiovascular disease (CVD), a set of pathologies commonly associated with obesity, people with moderate obesity exhibit a lower risk versus people in the normal weight

IntechOpen

BMI category [6]. This indicates that bodyweight recommendations are contradictory to mortality statistics. However, across a population level there is significantly increased hazard ratio for numerous diseases with increasing BMI, and obesity.

1.2 Adiposity and disease risk

The premise of BMI as a predictor of health-related outcomes is on the basis that it serves as a proxy for adiposity. However, BMI is a poor predictor of body fat since overall body weight is more dependent on lean mass [7]. Numerous studies have demonstrated that more direct measures of adiposity have a greater capacity than BMI to predict poor metabolic health outcomes and have potential in alternatively defining obesity [8–12]. In fact, these alternative metrics are often used by researchers investigating obesity because they better correlate with poor outcomes in instances where high BMI lacks correlation [13, 14]. BMI continues to be used consistently and ubiquitously in public and healthcare settings, but it is a crude predictor of disease risk, both due to its poor correlative value with adiposity, but also because of inconsistent correlations between disease and adiposity itself. Metabolic syndrome is

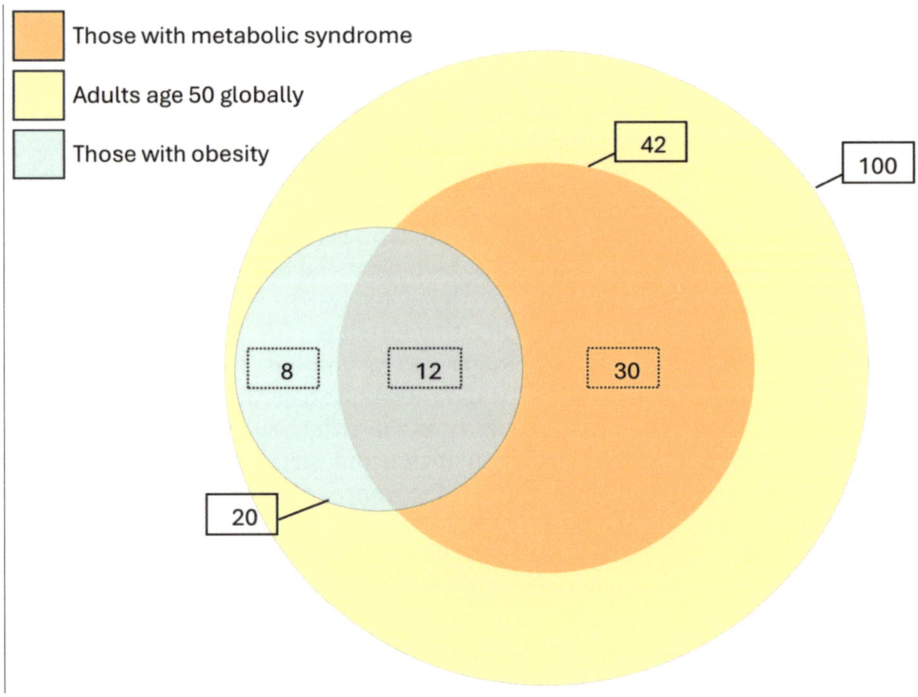

Figure 1.
People with obesity have a higher risk of metabolic syndrome, but the majority of people with metabolic syndrome do not have obesity. The numbers represented on the figure demonstrate the approximate prevalence of obesity and metabolic syndrome globally, taking age 50 as representative. The numbers are approximate and based on literature review – approximately 16% of adults globally have obesity [16], with those age 50 having approximately 1.2x higher rates [17, 18]. The overall rate of metabolic syndrome globally is approximately 30% across BMI categories, with 1.4x higher rates in those age 50 [19–21]. The rate of metabolic syndrome is higher in those with obesity (approximately 60% in people age 50) [19, 20, 22, 23]. The rate of metabolic syndrome in those without obesity (BMI < 30) across ages is approximately 25% overall, and approximately 38% for people age 50, but varies from 9 to 60% depending on the year of the study (as rates are increasing) defining criteria for metabolic syndrome (which sometimes dictate a high BMI), location of the study and the age profile of the cohort [22–25].

an indicator of adipose dysfunction and is measured using a number of clinical risk factors which together predict type 2 diabetes and CVD [15]. Both people with and without obesity are developing metabolic syndrome at increasing rates (**Figure 1**). Overall, this indicates that although quantification of adipose tissue, either directly or as an estimate using BMI, does associate with many health outcomes, this effect is likely due to a qualitative change in adipose function which is often associated with, but not dependent on a change in volume.

2. Adipose tissue function and dysfunction

2.1 Adipose tissue is a vital organ

The narrative of pathological adipose tissue has often been in describing its excess rather than its function and dysfunction. In focusing on reducing this excess, the vital functions of adipose as a bodily organ has been diminished. Adipose tissue is mostly regarded for its crucial role in survival by providing fuel in periods of low nutrient availability, and during pregnancy and lactation. This capacity of adipose tissue to handle, process and store fatty acids is also imperative to prevent lipotoxicity from fatty acids which must be stored safely but which are essential for the physiological functioning of every cell in the body. Adipose tissue is highly sensitive to metabolic, endocrine and immune changes, and responds by signalling to regulate numerous downstream physiologic functions. Distinct depots of adipose tissue have distinct functions, and have different relationships with metabolic health. Very broadly, adipose tissue can be categorised into visceral white adipose tissue (vWAT), subcutaneous white adipose tissue (sWAT) and brown adipose tissue (BAT). vWAT surrounds the viscera and its expansion is independently associated with those metabolic dysfunctions traditionally linked to obesity. sWAT is predominantly located in the upper legs and lower torso and its expansion is generally healthful and does not tend to associate with metabolic pathology. BAT contrasts with WAT and its volume negatively correlates with WAT volume. BAT is highly vascularised and dense in mitochondria, it serves to generate heat through inefficient metabolism. Some of the roles of each of these in health and disease are discussed in this book.

2.2 Physiologically relevant adipose dysfunction

Adipose dysfunction can occur with excess expansion, but is also recorded in cases without excess expansion and those with insufficient expansion. Interestingly, there are commonalities in the dysfunctions described in obesity and in underweight-associated adipose dysfunction indicating that both are associated with a disruption to the important functions performed by this tissue [26, 27].

3. Mediators of adipose dysfunction

3.1 Genetic and epigenetic contributions

There are both direct and indirect genetic contributions to adipogenic contributions to body weight, body shape and metabolic health, which can be dependent and independent of each other. A few rare genetic disorders such as the imprinted gene disorder Prader Willi syndrome are directly linked to a very high risk of central obesity (i.e. visceral adiposity). Outside of rare disorders, a larger number of genetic polymorphisms are associated with propensity toward more moderate risk phenotypes. Genetic and/or epigenetic modifications that alter gene expression can be associated with altered activity or feeding behaviours or food preference, others associated with whole-body metabolism and nutrient handling, while others are associated with physiological preference for which adipose depot expands in response to excess nutrition, additionally there are those modifications that alter susceptibility to obesogenic environmental stimuli [28–35].

3.2 The obesogenic environment

Discussions on the role of the environment in shaping adipose homeostasis primarily focusing on the "obesogenic" Western diet and lifestyle factors, such as exercise and access to green spaces [36–39]. As well as these important factors, numerous other aspects of the environment impact adipose tissue health. These factors are wide-ranging from sleep schedules to chemical exposure, and are often highly interlinked and confounding [40–43]. For example, gene environment interactions result in differential vulnerability to exposures [44–46]. Socioeconomic status also correlates with BMI in a manner dependent on geography [47]. Whether linked to lower or higher BMI, higher socioeconomic status tends to afford a level of protection from adipose dysfunction, disease incidence and negative outcomes via diverse modalities including type of employment, local pollution levels, access to medical supports, and access to suitable nutrition and exercise opportunities [48–53]. There are numerous compounds that we inadvertently handle and consume in our daily lives also known to cause adipose dysfunction and disrupt metabolism [42, 54, 55]. These health effects are associated with chronic low level exposure to these common compounds and environmental contaminants, many of which are lipophilic and bioaccumulate within bodily lipid stores [54, 56–58]. Exposures come from the contents of fire extinguishers, the non-stick coating on cookware, fragrances and air fresheners, fire-retardant coating on furniture, water-proof coating on clothing, cleaning products, cosmetics products, adhesives, and more [59–61]. These compounds are found in human tissues at levels that correlate with workplace and lifestyle-associated exposures – for example hairdressers and cleaners have higher burdens of compounds used in cosmetic and cleaning products respectively, while those compounds used in manufacturing plants and fire extinguishers are found at higher levels in people who work in factories and as firefighters respectively [62–66]. As well as direct exposure, these compounds are released into the environment during their use and build up in soil, water and air, they are taken up by plants which are then eaten by us and by the animals we eat, we drink them in our water supply, and we breath them in the air [60, 67]. The links between adipose dysfunction, metabolic health and disease risk demonstrate the importance of adipose tissue research for human health, and the role of the environment in mediating this indicates an important role of policy in reducing the burden of adipose-mediated ill health.

4. Conclusion

Adipose tissue dysfunction is increasing globally, and is associated with systemic metabolic dysfunction and disease risk, yet adipose tissue – the defining tissue of

DOI: http://dx.doi.org/10.5772/intechopen.1009588

metabolic dysfunction and obesity – is far from fully understood. Importantly for our understanding of aetiology and capacity for successful intervention, there are increasing rates of metabolic disorder in people with and without obesity. Therefore, focus of BMI as the major predictor of metabolic dysfunction, and of diet and lifestyle as the exclusive preventative intervention is handicapping efforts to improve metabolic health for more than a billion people worldwide. Improving our understanding of adipose tissue as a vital organ, and detailing the mechanisms by which it functions healthfully, and defining specific mechanisms of its dysfunction will be crucial for global public health as the number of people with adipose dysfunction continues to climb. As well as limiting success in improving health and wellbeing, the focus on BMI, diet and lifestyle places an undue onus on individuals for their own health status, including diagnoses that are commonly linked to obesity such as cancer. Instead identifying adipose dysfunction directly and targeting therapeutic development and interventions toward improving adipose tissue function could in the future yield better outcomes for those who stand to with the highest need, and therefore can benefit the most.

Author details

Féaron C. Cassidy[1,2]

1 Kathleen Lonsdale Institute for Human Health Research, Maynooth University, Maynooth, Co Kildare, Ireland

2 Department of Medicine Huddinge, Center for Infectious Medicine, Karolinska Institutet, Karolinska, Sweden

*Address all correspondence to: fearon.cassidy@mu.ie

IntechOpen

© 2025 The Author(s). Licensee IntechOpen. This chapter is distributed under the terms of the Creative Commons Attribution License (http://creativecommons.org/licenses/by/3.0), which permits unrestricted use, distribution, and reproduction in any medium, provided the original work is properly cited.

References

[1] Bhaskaran K, dos-Santos-Silva I, Leon DA, Douglas IJ, Smeeth L. Association of BMI with overall and cause-specific mortality: A population-based cohort study of 3·6 million adults in the UK. The Lancet Diabetes and Endocrinology. 2018;**6**(12):944-953. DOI: 10.1016/S2213-8587(18)30288-2

[2] Amy NK, Aalborg A, Lyons P, Keranen L. Barriers to routine gynecological cancer screening for White and African-American obese women. International Journal of Obesity. 2006;**30**(1):147-155. DOI: 10.1038/sj.ijo.0803105

[3] Cusimano MC, Simpson AN, Han A, Hayeems R, Bernardini MQ, Robertson D, et al. Barriers to care for women with low-grade endometrial cancer and morbid obesity: A qualitative study. BMJ Open. 2019;**9**(6):e026872. DOI: 10.1136/bmjopen-2018-026872

[4] Graham Y, Hayes C, Cox J, Mahawar K, Fox A, Yemm H. A systematic review of obesity as a barrier to accessing cancer screening services. Obesity Science and Practice. 2022;**8**(6):715-727. DOI: 10.1002/OSP4.606

[5] Wee CW, McCarthy EP, Davis RB, Phillips RS. Screening for cervical and breast cancer: Is obesity an unrecognized barrier to preventive care? Annals of Internal Medicine. 2000;**132**(9):697-704. DOI: 10.7326/0003-4819-132-9-200005020-00003

[6] Owusu Adjah ES, Ray KK, Paul SK. Ethnicity-specific association of BMI levels at diagnosis of type 2 diabetes with cardiovascular disease and all-cause mortality risk. Acta Diabetologica. 2019;**56**(1):87-96. DOI: 10.1007/s00592-018-1219-7

[7] Romero-Corral A, Somers VK, Sierra-Johnson J, Thomas RJ, Collazo-Clavell ML, Korinek J, et al. Accuracy of body mass index in diagnosing obesity in the adult general population. International Journal of Obesity. 2008;**32**(6). DOI: 10.1038/ijo.2008.11

[8] Bi X, Tey SL, Leong C, Quek R, Loo YT, Henry CJ. Correlation of adiposity indices with cardiovascular disease risk factors in healthy adults of Singapore: A cross-sectional study. BMC Obesity. 2016;**3**(1):33. DOI: 10.1186/s40608-016-0114-4

[9] O'Connor KG, Harman SM, Stevens TE, Jayme JJ, Bellantoni MF, Busby-Whitehead MJ, et al. Interrelationship of spontaneous growth hormone axis activity, body fat, and serum lipids is healthy elderly women and men. Metabolism. 1999;**48**(11):1424-1431. DOI: 10.1016/S0026-0495(99)90154-3

[10] Ofstad AP, Sommer C, Birkeland KI, Bjørgaas MR, Gran JM, Gulseth HL, et al. Comparison of the associations between non-traditional and traditional indices of adiposity and cardiovascular mortality: An observational study of one million person-years of follow-up. International Journal of Obesity. 2019;**43**(5):1082-1092. DOI: 10.1038/s41366-019-0353-9

[11] Raheem J, Sliz E, Shin J, Holmes MV, Pike GB, Richer L, et al. Visceral adiposity is associated with metabolic profiles predictive of type 2 diabetes and myocardial infarction. Communications Medicine. 2022;**2**(1):81. DOI: 10.1038/S43856-022-00140-5

[12] Wang B, Necheles J, Ouyang F, Ma W, Li Z, Liu X, et al. Monozygotic

co-twin analyses of body composition measurements and serum lipids. Preventive Medicine. 2007;**45**(5):358-365. DOI: 10.1016/j.ypmed.2007.07.014

[13] Ahn S, Han K, Lee J-E, Jeun S-S, Park Y-M, Yang SH. Associations of general and abdominal obesity with the risk of glioma development. Cancers. 2021;**13**(12):2859. DOI: 10.3390/cancers13122859

[14] Barbi J, Patnaik SK, Pabla S, Zollo R, Smith RJ, Sass SN, et al. Visceral obesity promotes lung cancer progression—Toward resolution of the obesity paradox in lung cancer. Journal of Thoracic Oncology. 2021;**16**(8):1333-1348. DOI: 10.1016/j.jtho.2021.04.020

[15] Kassi E, Pervanidou P, Kaltsas G, Chrousos G. Metabolic syndrome: Definitions and controversies. BMC Medicine. 2011;**9**(1):48. DOI: 10.1186/1741-7015-9-48

[16] Ezzati M. Worldwide Trends in Underweight and Obesity from 1990 to 2022: A Pooled Analysis of 3663 Population-Representative Studies with 222 Million Children, Adolescents, and Adults NCD Risk Factor Collaboration (NCD-RisC)*. 2024. DOI: 10.1016/S0140-6736(23)02750-2

[17] Emmerich SD, Fryar CD, Stierman B, Ogden CL. Obesity and Severe Obesity Prevalence in Adults: United States, August 2021–August 2023 Key Findings Data from the National Health and Nutrition Examination Survey. 2021. Available from: https://www.cdc.gov/nchs/products/index.htm

[18] Reed B, Abunnaja S. The epidemiology of obesity. Handbook of Metabolic and Bariatric Surgery. 2023:20-26. DOI: 10.1002/9781119521686.ch3

[19] Damiri B, Abualsoud MS, Samara AM, Salameh SK. Metabolic syndrome among overweight and obese adults in Palestinian refugee camps. Diabetology and Metabolic Syndrome. 2018;**10**(1):34. DOI: 10.1186/s13098-018-0337-2

[20] Engin A. The definition and prevalence of obesity and metabolic syndrome. In: Advances in Experimental Medicine and Biology. Vol. 960. 2017. DOI: 10.1007/978-3-319-48382-5_1

[21] Noubiap JJ, Nansseu JR, Lontchi-Yimagou E, Nkeck JR, Nyaga UF, Ngouo AT, et al. Geographic distribution of metabolic syndrome and its components in the general adult population: A meta-analysis of global data from 28 million individuals. Diabetes Research and Clinical Practice. 2022;**188**:109924. DOI: 10.1016/j.diabres.2022.109924

[22] Mata A, Jasul G, Jr. Prevalence of metabolic syndrome and its individual features across different (Normal, overweight, pre-obese and obese) body mass index (BMI) categories in a tertiary hospital in the Philippines. Journal of the ASEAN Federation of Endocrine Societies. 2017;**32**(2):117-122. DOI: 10.15605/jafes.032.02.04

[23] Shi TH, Wang B, Natarajan S. The influence of metabolic syndrome in predicting mortality risk among US adults: Importance of metabolic syndrome even in adults with normal weight. Preventing Chronic Disease. 2020;**17**:200020. DOI: 10.5888/pcd17.200020

[24] Pluta W, Dudzińska W, Lubkowska A. Metabolic obesity in people with normal body weight (MONW)—Review of diagnostic criteria. International Journal of Environmental Research and Public Health. 2022;**19**(2):624. DOI: 10.3390/ijerph19020624

[25] Wildman RP. The obese without Cardiometabolic risk factor clustering and the normal weight with cardiometabolic risk factor clustering. Archives of Internal Medicine. 2008;**168**(15):1617. DOI: 10.1001/archinte.168.15.1617

[26] Joseph A, Chen H, Anagnostopoulos G, Montégut L, Lafarge A, Motiño O, et al. Effects of acyl-coenzyme A binding protein (ACBP)/diazepam-binding inhibitor (DBI) on body mass index. Cell Death and Disease. 2021;**12**(6):599. DOI: 10.1038/s41419-021-03864-9

[27] Soeters MR, Soeters PB. The evolutionary benefit of insulin resistance. Clinical Nutrition. 2012;**31**(6):1002-1007. DOI: 10.1016/j.clnu.2012.05.011

[28] Fall T, Ingelsson E. Genome-wide association studies of obesity and metabolic syndrome. Molecular and Cellular Endocrinology. 2014;**382**(1):740-757. DOI: 10.1016/j.mce.2012.08.018

[29] Ghosh S, Bouchard C. Convergence between biological, behavioural and genetic determinants of obesity. Nature Reviews Genetics. 2017;**18**(12):731-748. DOI: 10.1038/nrg.2017.72

[30] Lindgren CM, Heid IM, Randall JC, Lamina C, Steinthorsdottir V, Qi L, et al. Genome-wide association scan meta-analysis identifies three loci influencing adiposity and fat distribution. PLoS Genetics. 2009;**5**(6):e1000508. DOI: 10.1371/journal.pgen.1000508

[31] Moyerbrailean GA, Richards AL, Kurtz D, Kalita CA, Davis GO, Harvey CT, et al. High-throughput allele-specific expression across 250 environmental conditions. Genome Research. 2016;**26**(12):1627-1638. DOI: 10.1101/gr.209759.116

[32] Ndiaye FK, Huyvaert M, Ortalli A, Canouil M, Lecoeur C, Verbanck M, et al. The expression of genes in top obesity-associated loci is enriched in insula and substantia nigra brain regions involved in addiction and reward. International Journal of Obesity. 2020;**44**(2):539-543. DOI: 10.1038/s41366-019-0428-7

[33] Pan DZ, Miao Z, Comenho C, Rajkumar S, Koka A, Lee SHT, et al. Identification of TBX15 as an adipose master trans regulator of abdominal obesity genes. Genome Medicine. 2021;**13**(1):123. DOI: 10.1186/s13073-021-00939-2

[34] Pledger SL, Ahmadizar F. Gene-environment interactions and the effect on obesity risk in low and middle-income countries: A scoping review. Frontiers in Endocrinology. 2023;**14**. DOI: 10.3389/fendo.2023.1230445

[35] Shungin D, Winkler TW, Croteau-Chonka DC, Ferreira T, Locke AE, Mägi R, et al. New genetic loci link adipose and insulin biology to body fat distribution. Nature. 2015;**518**(7538):187-196. DOI: 10.1038/nature14132

[36] de Albuquerque FM, Pessoa MC, Filgueiras MDS, do Carmo AS, Vegi ASF, Ribeiro AQ, et al. Neighborhood obesogenic environment and cardiometabolic risk in Brazilian children: The mediation role of the mother's body mass index. American Journal of Human Biology. 2023;**35**(3). DOI: 10.1002/ajhb.23835

[37] Fisberg M, Maximino P, Kain J, Kovalskys I. Obesogenic environment – Intervention opportunities. Jornal de Pediatria (Versão Em Português). 2016;**92**(3):S30-S39. DOI: 10.1016/j.jpedp.2016.03.018

[38] Jia P. Obesogenic environment and childhood obesity. Obesity Reviews.

2021;**22**(S1):e13158. DOI: 10.1111/obr.13158

[39] Swinburn B, Egger G, Raza F. Dissecting obesogenic environments: The development and application of a framework for identifying and prioritizing environmental interventions for obesity. Preventive Medicine. 1999;**29**(6):563-570. DOI: 10.1006/pmed.1999.0585

[40] de Bont J, Márquez S, Fernández-Barrés S, Warembourg C, Koch S, Persavento C, et al. Urban environment and obesity and weight-related behaviours in primary school children. Environment International. 2021;**155**:106700. DOI: 10.1016/j.envint.2021.106700

[41] Kamel Boulos MN, Koh K. Smart city lifestyle sensing, big data, geo-analytics and intelligence for smarter public health decision-making in overweight, obesity and type 2 diabetes prevention: The research we should be doing. International Journal of Health Geographics. 2021;**20**(1):12. DOI: 10.1186/s12942-021-00266-0

[42] Martínez-Esquivel A, Trujillo-Silva DJ, Cilia-López VG. Impact of environmental pollution on the obesogenic environment. Nutrition Reviews. 2022;**80**(7):1787-1799. DOI: 10.1093/nutrit/nuac003

[43] Masood B, Moorthy M. Causes of obesity: A review. Clinical Medicine. 2023;**23**(4):284-291. DOI: 10.7861/clinmed.2023-0168

[44] Aulsebrook LC, Wong BBM, Hall MD. Can pharmaceutical pollution alter the spread of infectious disease? A case study using fluoxetine. Philosophical Transactions of the Royal Society B: Biological Sciences. 2023;**378**(1873). DOI: 10.1098/rstb.2022.0010

[45] Parajuli RP, Goodrich JM, Chan HM, Lemire M, Ayotte P, Hegele RA, et al. Variation in biomarker levels of metals, persistent organic pollutants, and omega-3 fatty acids in association with genetic polymorphisms among Inuit in Nunavik, Canada. Environmental Research. 2021;**200**:11393. DOI: 10.1016/j.envres.2021.111393

[46] Zhu H, Kartiko S, Finnell RH. Importance of gene–environment interactions in the etiology of selected birth defects. Clinical Genetics. 2009;**75**(5):409-423. DOI: 10.1111/j.1399-0004.2009.01174.x

[47] Cassidy FC, Lafferty S, Coleman CM. The role of gender in the onset, development and impact of type 2 diabetes mellitus and its Co-morbidities. In: Type 2 Diabetes - From Pathophysiology to Cyber Systems. London, UK: IntechOpen; 2021. DOI: 10.5772/intechopen.94271

[48] Bancks MP, Kershaw K, Carson AP, Gordon-Larsen P, Schreiner PJ, Carnethon MR. Association of modifiable risk factors in young adulthood with racial disparity in incident type 2 diabetes during middle adulthood. JAMA. 2017;**318**(24):2457. DOI: 10.1001/jama.2017.19546

[49] Bansal E, Placidi D, Carver S, Renzetti S, Giorgino A, Cagna G, et al. Metabolic outcomes in southern Italian preadolescents residing near an industrial complex: The role of residential location and socioeconomic status. International Journal of Environmental Research and Public Health. 2019;**16**(11):2036. DOI: 10.3390/ijerph16112036

[50] Conway BN, Han X, Munro HM, Gross AL, Shu X-O, Hargreaves MK, et al. The obesity epidemic and rising diabetes incidence in a low-income racially diverse southern US cohort.

PLoS One. 2018;**13**(1):e0190993. DOI: 10.1371/journal.pone.0190993

[51] Johnson KA, Jones-Smith J, Curriero FC, Cheskin LJ, Benjamin-Neelon SE, Perin J, et al. Low-income black and hispanic children's neighborhood food environments and weight trajectories in early childhood. Academic Pediatrics. 2020;**20**(6):784-792. DOI: 10.1016/j.acap.2019.11.013

[52] Roberts DE. Fatal Invention: How Science, Politics, and Big Business Re-Create Race in the Twenty-First Century. New York City: New Press; 2011

[53] VoPham T, Kim NJ, Berry K, Mendoza JA, Kaufman JD, Ioannou GN. PM2.5 air pollution exposure and nonalcoholic fatty liver disease in the Nationwide inpatient Sample. Environmental Research. 2022;**213**:113611. DOI: 10.1016/j.envres.2022.113611

[54] Jackson E, Shoemaker R, Larian N, Cassis L. Adipose tissue as a site of toxin accumulation. Comprehensive Physiology. 2017;7(4):1085-1135. DOI: 10.1002/cphy.c160038

[55] Sun J, Fang R, Wang H, Xu D-X, Yang J, Huang X, et al. A review of environmental metabolism disrupting chemicals and effect biomarkers associating disease risks: Where exposomics meets metabolomics. Environment International. 2022;**158**:106941. DOI: 10.1016/j.envint.2021.106941

[56] Covaci A, de Boer J, Ryan JJ, Voorspoels S, Schepens P. Distribution of organobrominated and organochlorinated contaminants in Belgian human adipose tissue. Environmental Research. 2002;**88**(3):210-218. DOI: 10.1006/enrs.2002.4334

[57] Power A, White P, McHugh B, Berrow S, Schlingermann M, Tannian M, et al. Persistent pollutants in northern gannet Morus bassanus eggs in Ireland: Levels and colony differences. Environmental Pollution. 2021;**268**:115723. DOI: 10.1016/j.envpol.2020.115723

[58] Schrenk D, Bignami M, Bodin L, Chipman JK, del Mazo J, Grasl-Kraupp B, et al. Risk to human health related to the presence of perfluoroalkyl substances in food. EFSA Journal. 2020;**18**(9). DOI: 10.2903/j.efsa.2020.6223

[59] Gibson G, Cundy A, Kafwamfwa N, Stewart A. "Old" and "new" contaminants and their management: Learning from the past, looking to the future. Environmental Geochemistry and Health. 2023;**45**(4):1091-1105. DOI: 10.1007/s10653-021-01042-6

[60] Laws EA. Aquatic Pollution, an Introductory Text. 2nd ed. New York City: John Wiley & Sons, Inc; 1993

[61] Steinemann A. Ten questions concerning air fresheners and indoor built environments. Building and Environment. 2017;**111**:279-284. DOI: 10.1016/j.buildenv.2016.11.009

[62] Eneh OC. Health effects of selected trace elements in hairdressing cosmetics on hairdressers in Enugu, Nigeria. Scientific Reports. 2021;**11**(1):20352. DOI: 10.1038/s41598-021-00022-1

[63] Himani KR, Ansari JA, Mahdi AA, Sharma D, Karunanand B, Datta SK. Blood Lead levels in occupationally exposed workers involved in battery factories of Delhi-NCR region: Effect on vitamin D and calcium metabolism. Indian Journal of Clinical Biochemistry. 2020;**35**(1):80-87. DOI: 10.1007/s12291-018-0797-z

[64] Johansson GM, Jönsson BAG, Axmon A, Lindh CH, Lind M-L, Gustavsson M, et al. Exposure of hairdressers to ortho- and meta-toluidine in hair dyes. Occupational and Environmental Medicine. 2015;**72**(1):57-63. DOI: 10.1136/oemed-2013-101960

[65] Rosenfeld PE, Spaeth KR, Remy LL, Byers V, Muerth SA, Hallman RC, et al. Perfluoroalkyl substances exposure in firefighters: Sources and implications. Environmental Research. 2023;**220**:115164. DOI: 10.1016/j.envres.2022.115164

[66] Wu C-F, Peng C-Y, Liu C-C, Lin W-Y, Pan C-H, Cheng C-M, et al. Ambient melamine exposure and urinary biomarkers of early renal injury. Journal of the American Society of Nephrology. 2015;**26**(11):2821-2829. DOI: 10.1681/ASN.2014121233

[67] Ankley GT, Cureton P, Hoke RA, Houde M, Kumar A, Kurias J, et al. Assessing the ecological risks of per- and polyfluoroalkyl substances: Current state-of-the science and a proposed path forward. Environmental Toxicology and Chemistry. 2020;**40**(3):564-605. DOI: 10.1002/etc.4869

Section 2

White Adipose Tissue Homeostasis in Health and Disease

Chapter 2

Adipose Tissue and Cancer

Noor Bakour, Claudine Duggan and Stephanie L. Annett

Abstract

White adipose tissue (WAT) is a major endocrine organ with crucial physiological functions in energy homeostasis, hormonal regulation, and immune function. It is comprised of a vast repertoire of cell types including adipocytes, fibroblasts, immune cells, endothelial cells, and stem cells each with their own tissue-specific role. Disturbances in AT physiology can occur in conditions such as metabolic syndrome and obesity and are associated with the development of several non-communicable diseases including cancer. Cancer is a leading cause of death globally, and alarmingly, rates of both cancer and obesity are rising. Obesity has become a well-established risk factor for the development of several cancer types and can lead to worse outcomes and increased mortality rates in patients with cancer. Dysfunctional AT associated with obesity demonstrates an altered cell composition profile and secretes factors that benefit cellular transformation, cancer growth and progression, and metastasis. In addition, a bidirectional relationship between the AT and cancer cells involves cell-cell crosstalk, which ultimately benefits tumor growth. Here, we discuss the epidemiology of obesity-associated cancer and the molecular mechanisms that link AT dysfunction in obesity to the development and progression of cancer.

Keywords: cancer, adipose tissue, obesity, cancer risk, tumor development, cancer progression, cancer-associated adipocyte

1. Introduction

Adipose tissue (AT) in mammals is comprised of three distinct types, namely white adipose tissue (WAT), brown AT, and beige AT, which are characterized by their functions. For the purpose of this chapter, we will focus on WAT, herein referred to as AT, whose contribution to cancer has been best characterized. Similarly, the term adipocyte hereafter specifically refers to white adipocytes. Although once considered an inert tissue that was solely responsible for insulating other organs, WAT is now recognized as the primary energy store for the body and is essential for maintaining systemic metabolic homeostasis. Furthermore, in conjunction with other tissue-resident cells of the AT, adipocytes are increasingly gaining recognition for their modulation and regulation of inflammatory, metabolic, and endocrine processes. However, in conditions such as obesity, the composition and function of the AT can become altered, which can affect local tissue environments, as well as produce systemic effects.

Obesity is a chronic medical condition characterized by the presence of excess AT and is generally defined medically as a Body Mass Index (BMI) of ≥30. From a global

IntechOpen

health perspective, obesity is an exponentially growing problem and has reached epidemic proportions in geographical regions such as North America, Europe, and Australia/New Zealand. The World Health Organization (WHO) estimates that up to 67% of adults live with overweight or obesity (BMI >25 and ≥ 30, respectively) in the regions of highest prevalence which include the Americas and Europe [1, 2]. Within the last three decades, obesity prevalence has steadily increased. This is particularly concerning considering that obesity is a major risk factor for multiple non-communicable diseases, including Type 2 Diabetes Mellitus (T2DM), cardiovascular diseases, and certain cancers, posing both health and economic implications within the impacted regions.

Individuals who are categorized as having overweight or obesity are now considered to have a significantly greater risk of developing cancer, with an estimated 3.9% of all cancer cases globally linked to these conditions [3]. Cancer incidence is increasing among the global population and it is estimated that one in three persons will develop cancer over their lifetime. There were approximately 19.9 million cases of cancer diagnosed worldwide in 2022 according to the World Health Organization's (WHO) Global Cancer Observatory statistics [4]. Although there have been major advances in the treatment of many cancers, it remains one of the leading causes of death annually, particularly in European and North American populations where it has been reported to account for approximately one in six deaths [5]. Many epidemiological studies have documented a relationship between excess adiposity and cancer incidence with a causal relationship established for 13 cancer types by the International Agency for Research on Cancer (IARC) in 2016 (**Table 1**) [19].

Given the known associations of several cancer types with obesity and increased BMI, current obesity trends are worrying and pose a risk of continuing disease burden. Over the last 20 years, there has been a significant rise in both cancer-related

Cancer type	Relative risk of the highest BMI measured versus normal BMI	References
Corpus Uteri	7.1 (6.3–8.1)	[6]
Esophageal adenocarcinoma	4.8 (3.0–7.7)	[7]
Renal Cell	1.8 (1.7–1.9)	[8]
Gastric cardia	1.8 (1.3–2.5)	[9]
Liver	1.8 (1.6–2.1)	[10]
Gallbladder	1.6 (1.5–1.8)	[11]
Meningioma	1.5 (1.3–1.8)	[12]
Pancreas	1.5 (1.2–1.8)	[13]
Multiple Myeloma	1.5 (1.2–2.0)	[14]
Colorectal	1.3 (1.3–1.4)	[15]
Breast (postmenopausal)	1.1 (1.1–1.2)	[16]
Ovary	1.1 (1.1–1.2)	[17]
Thyroid	1.1 (1.0–1.1)	[18]

Source: Adapted from [19].

Table 1.
List of cancers with established associations with obesity and the relative risk of cancer onset with increased BMI.

deaths and disability-adjusted life years related specifically to high BMI [20, 21]. A long-term study spanning the period from 1990 to 2019 estimated a 160% increase in cancer-related deaths attributed to high BMI specifically [20]. These high BMI-related cancer incidences and/or morbidities affect various populations differently with East Asian, European, and North American populations displaying the highest incidence of obesity-associated cancers. In terms of gender differences, women are predominantly affected by high BMI-associated cancers by approximately two-fold compared to men [22]. Evidence of this link from epidemiological studies is further supported by experimental studies using animal models of obesity. Although these are unable to fully recapitulate the exact physiological conditions that occur in humans with obesity in many cases, various *in vivo* models including diet-induced and genetic models of obesity have been shown to drive the progression of multiple cancer types, as reviewed in the work of Lee [23]. Due to the global health burden of obesity, much of the current research is focused on its association with cancer. Indeed, there are some cancer types for which low BMI (<18.5 kg/m^2 or underweight) is a risk factor, potentially also further implicating the AT in the development of certain cancer types although in a contrasting manner. This is evident in several cancer types including lung cancer and esophageal squamous cell carcinoma [24, 25].

It is clear from both epidemiological and experimental perspectives that there are strong correlations between BMI and cancer development/progression. Here we discuss the mechanisms that link the two conditions with a specific focus on the role of the AT and the implications and future perspective of cancer therapy in this context.

2. The role of AT in influencing cancer growth and progression

2.1 Changes to AT composition and function in obesity

AT is composed of a variety of cell types, with adipocytes accounting for between 40 and 50% of the cell population in healthy tissues. The remaining cells comprise the stromal-vascular fraction (SVF) of AT, which contains immune cells, endothelial cells, and stromal cells [26, 27]. Adipocytes serve as the primary energy store for the body and are essential for maintaining systemic metabolic homeostasis. In response to increased energy, adipocytes can increase their cell mass, allowing triglycerides to accumulate, which can later be harnessed for energy when required [28]. Furthermore, AT can influence insulin resistance and sensitivity, angiogenesis, lipid metabolism, and inflammation by secreting factors such as free fatty acids (FFA), pro-inflammatory cytokines, and adipokines in exosomes [29–32].

Typically, normal AT-associated processes are tightly regulated. However, in obesity, the composition and function of AT can become altered; AT expansion occurs as a result of adipocyte hypertrophy (increased cell mass) and hyperplasia (increased proliferation of progenitor cells) [33, 34]. Compared to most lean individuals, the AT of individuals with obesity is commonly associated with a dysregulated inflammatory phenotype and can be characterized by increased immune cell infiltration into its stromal compartments. The consequences of these changes affect the local AT microenvironment but also have systemic effects. Dysregulated adipocytes demonstrate increased secretion of growth factors as well as pro-inflammatory cytokines and adipokines (cytokines produced specifically by adipocytes). In addition, mitochondrial dysfunction and cell death rates increase [35–37]. Angiogenesis becomes insufficient in obesity-associated AT dysfunction, leading to a hypoxic environment [38].

Together, these tissue changes can create favorable conditions for carcinogenesis and provide essential biomolecules for malignancies to grow and evolve.

2.2 Obesity-associated AT inflammation and cancer

Healthy AT hosts a unique immune cell repertoire, which has key roles in maintaining tissue homeostasis and mediating immune responses. Adipocytes and AT-resident immune cells secrete pro- and anti-inflammatory cytokines, which mount and resolve inflammatory responses [39, 40]. However, such homeostasis can become lost in obesity, and instead, a characteristic state of chronic low-grade inflammation prevails in these instances. Chronic inflammation is a well-recognized cancer risk factor and represents a Hallmark of Cancer, i.e., a biological characteristic that favors tumor cell survival, growth, and metastasis [41, 42]. Several studies have highlighted systemic inflammation as a risk factor for cancers such as colorectal and lung cancers [43, 44]. This relationship is further supported by the existence of several cancer types that are associated with chronic infections and inflammation (e.g., *Helicobacter pylori* and gastric cancer, human papillomavirus (HPV) and cervical cancer, inflammatory bowel disease, and colorectal cancer). Furthermore, one study investigating the relationship between obesity and colorectal cancer survival and progression posited that obesity-associated inflammation was a greater risk factor for cancer progression and mortality than obesity itself [45]. The initial triggers of the cascade resulting in chronic inflammation in obesity characterized by AT dysfunction are not yet fully clear. However, increased infiltration of pro-inflammatory immune cells into obese AT, particularly pro-inflammatory macrophages, may at least partially play a role [46].

Studies in the early 2000s provided the first evidence that the degree of adiposity can influence the composition of the AT immune cell repertoire. In lean humans and mice, approximately 5% of immune cells within AT are tissue-resident macrophages. However, this can increase to as much as 40–50% in obesity [47–49]. In addition, numbers of anti-inflammatory regulatory T cells (Tregs) decrease in obesity, while infiltrations of $CD8^+$ T-cells and $CD4^+$ T_H1 cells increase, further contributing to an inflammatory tissue microenvironment [50–54].

The tissue-resident macrophages within dysfunctional AT further contribute to inflammation by adopting a pro-inflammatory phenotype. AT from lean mice has been shown to possess tissue-resident macrophages that are more likely to be M2-polarized, promoting tissue remodeling and anti-inflammatory cytokine secretion. However, in obese mice, pro-inflammatory M1 macrophages are abundant and contribute to an inflamed tissue microenvironment [55]. These high infiltrations of macrophages surround necrotic adipocytes to form inflammatory foci known as crown-like structures (CLS) [56–58]. Here, they become exposed to FFAs released during obesity-associated lipolysis. These FFAs can then bind to and activate toll-like receptor 4 (TLR4) expressed on the surface of these macrophages [59–62] The downstream inflammatory nuclear factor kappa-light-chain-enhancer of activated B cells (NF-κB) pathway is initiated and leads to transcription of pro-inflammatory genes such as cyclooxygenase-2 (COX-2), interleukin-1β (IL-1β), and tumor necrosis factor-α (TNFα) [59, 62], further perpetuating local and systemic inflammation. In addition, increased circulating insulin levels commonly observed in obesity can cause adipocytes to express chemokine ligand 2 (CCL2) [63]. CCL2 recruits macrophages to the AT where they can result in further CCL2 secretion, enabling pro-inflammatory macrophages to persist within the AT. These activated macrophages secrete pro-inflammatory factors such as TNFα, inducible nitric oxide synthase (iNOS), IL-1β, and IL-6, and also express pro-angiogenic factors which were shown to support tumor growth in mouse and human breast tissues [64, 65].

Along with altered immune cell composition within adipose depots, obesity is commonly associated with impaired immune cell functions [66]. This is supported by studies demonstrating increased susceptibility to infectious illness in individuals with obesity compared to lean individuals (reviewed in the work of Falagas and Kompoti [67]). For example, one study showed impaired immune cell function and increased secretion of the immunosuppressive cytokine IL-10 in dendritic cells from individuals with obesity compared to lean individuals [68]. However, it is noteworthy that some studies have shown opposite findings [69].

Similar to the increased infiltration of immune cells observed in dysfunctional AT, immune cell infiltration is a characteristic of most tumor types, and these immune cell infiltrates can play paradoxical roles in tumor progression in a context-dependent manner. Classically, the belief that immune cells serve to eradicate incipient tumors before they can progress prevailed. However, increasing evidence has shown that the inflammatory responses caused by these infiltrates can benefit tumors. For example, inflammation can provide growth factors and pro-angiogenic factors to the tumor microenvironment (TME). In addition, inflammatory signaling pathways such as NF-κB and signal transducer and activator of transcription factor 3 (STAT3) can stimulate cancer cell proliferation and promote cancer cell survival, providing a mechanistic link between obesity-associated inflammation and cancer [70, 71]. These pathways have also been suggested to play roles in epithelial-to-mesenchymal transition (EMT), as well as contributing to genomic instability by increasing DNA damage and disrupting DNA repair mechanisms [72]. These pathways can become constitutively activated in cancer via chronic exposure to inflammatory stimuli [73].

2.3 The role of AT insulin resistance in cancer

The links between AT and cancer are thought to be multifactorial and involve a complex interplay between several signaling pathways and physiological processes. Insulin resistance (IR) is a common condition in people with obesity, broadly characterized as an impairment in glucose uptake and utilization in response to insulin. IR can also be present in metabolically unhealthy lean individuals and potentially increase their risk of developing associated co-morbidities such as cancer [74, 75].

Insulin secreted by pancreatic β-cells enters the circulation and acts upon peripheral tissues to regulate carbohydrate, lipid, and protein metabolism within the body. Under normal physiological conditions, insulin acts upon the AT to regulate glucose uptake and promote triglyceride production from circulating FFAs while simultaneously inhibiting triglyceride hydrolysis [76]. Insulin resistance and AT dysfunction are tightly correlated. Hypertrophied adipocytes exceed their capacity for lipid storage and increase their rate of lipolysis, increasing the availability of FFAs and glucose, thus bypassing the regulatory functions of insulin [77, 78]. This may in turn promote insulin resistance in other tissues and organs, such as the liver, further exacerbating this systemic effect.

Cancer cells are known to reprogram their metabolism to meet the increased energy demands required for their rapid growth and division, and to adapt to nutrient availability within the TME. When necessary, they can upregulate *de novo* fatty acid synthesis to overcome nutrient barriers within this environment. However, they can also take up environmental FFAs for the same purpose and may harness the FFAs made available systemically and locally as a consequence of AT insulin resistance. Some tumors positioned adjacent to AT deposits, for example breast and prostate, may be particularly influenced by this phenomenon due to their proximity to the site of FFA production. CD36 (also known as fatty acid translocase) is a FA transporter that facilitates the uptake of extracellular FAs into cells for use in fatty acid oxidation (FAO). It is expressed by adipocytes as well as by many different cancers including breast, ovarian, brain, and gastric and has been implicated in their metastatic spread [79–82]. It has been reported that exposure of ovarian cancer cell lines to omental adipocytes induces the expression of CD36 and the subsequent uptake of FAs, leading to lipid accumulation in these cancer cells [80]. Additionally, an adipocyte-induced metastatic phenotype in ovarian cancer cells is abrogated through the inhibition of CD36 signaling, implicating the receptor directly in driving metastasis via FA uptake [80]. Similar functions for CD36 have been described in gastric cancer where the receptor was shown to facilitate palmitate acid-induced metastasis via the AKT/GSK-3β/β-catenin pathway in gastric cancer cell lines [82]. In breast cancer its expression has been reported to be required for anti-HER2 therapy resistance [81]. Other cellular components of the TME may also adapt to nutrient availability accordingly, facilitating tumor growth and metastasis. CD36 expression in macrophage populations is associated with obesity [83] while tumor-associated macrophages (TAMs) have been shown to express high levels of CD36 [84]. CD36 macrophage-specific knockout mice demonstrate significantly attenuated liver metastasis *in vivo* [84]. Furthermore, $CD36^+$ cancer-associated fibroblasts (CAFs) have been identified as inducers of a myeloid-derived suppressor cell phenotype in hepatic tumors and central to anti-PD-1 therapy resistance in *in vivo* models of hepatocellular carcinoma (HCC) [85].

2.4 Endocrine function of AT in cancer

AT is considered the largest endocrine organ of the body. To date, an AT secretome composed of over 50 different cytokines, adipokines, and steroid hormones has been characterized [86]. These molecules have many functions, including serving as mediators of innate immune responses and maintaining energy homeostasis. In addition to their endocrine functions, they can exert their functions in both autocrine and paracrine fashions [87, 88]. In conditions such as obesity, the normal secretory patterns of these factors from the AT can be disrupted, and the resulting consequences on endocrine signaling may favor the development and progression of multiple cancer types.

2.4.1 Estrogen signaling

Estrogens are a group of steroid hormones that consist of three major family members: estrone (E1), estradiol (E2), and estriol (E3). They are primarily produced by the female reproductive system in the pre-menopausal setting and regulate reproductive system development and secondary sex characteristics in females. E2 is the predominant form of the estrogens produced which signals via the classical estrogen receptor-α (ER) signaling pathway involving the translocation of the substrate-receptor complex from the cytoplasm to the nucleus where the receptor engages in DNA binding and transcription of estrogen-regulated genes.

The AT has a complex biological relationship with estrogen signaling. The normal physiology of the AT is regulated by estrogen but it is also responsible for the production of large amounts of estrogen itself. Estrogen is known to regulate AT tissue expansion with specific roles in adipocyte differentiation and proliferation [89, 90]. Gender-specific differences in its production highlight the protective role it has in terms of obesity. A high level of estrogen, for example in pre-menopausal women, promotes the deposition of subcutaneous AT, predominantly in the lower body which is protective from metabolic dysfunction. However, in those with lower estrogen levels, for example most men as well as postmenopausal women, deposition is instead predominantly around the viscera, which drives inflammation and insulin resistance [91, 92].

Changes in estrogen production and the related changes to AT composition bear particular importance in relation to breast cancer. ER-positive breast cancers represent the largest proportion of all breast cancer cases that occur annually and blockade of ER signaling is the primary molecular therapeutic intervention for this breast cancer subtype. Estrogen can signal through the ER to potentiate both genomic and non-genomic actions, regulating many pathways responsible for driving cellular growth, proliferation, EMT, and metastasis in cancer, as well as influencing non-cancer cells within the TME to support tumor growth [93]. Once ligand bound, the ER is translocated to the nucleus where it acts as a transcription factor, upregulating the expression of many genes with oncogenic potential. Estrogen can also have non-genomic effects, activating cytosolic-membrane bound ER or alternative receptors (such as the G-protein coupled estrogen receptor) to activate intracellular pathways that promote cellular growth and proliferation [94, 95].

Due to the positive correlation observed between adiposity and estrogen synthesis, it is thought that breast cancer development is driven via an increase in local estrogen production within the breast AT. However, systemic increases in estrogen levels have also been correlated with both BMI and cancer development [96]. Estrogen levels are often elevated in people with obesity due to an increase in aromatase enzyme expression within the AT, aromatase being the key enzyme responsible for the conversion of androgens to estrogen [97]. Increased secretion of factors such as TNFα, IL-6, and leptin that result from AT dysfunction can directly upregulate aromatase expression in both adipocyte and fibroblast populations within the AT [98–100]. In the case of breast cancer, several studies suggest that AT-resident fibroblasts or stromal cells are particularly important for this over-production of estrogen and may in fact contribute to endocrine therapy resistance in this manner [101]. Interestingly, adiponectin, which is negatively correlated with BMI, can inhibit induced aromatase expression in AT stromal fractions strengthening the association of obesity with breast cancer risk [100].

Although best characterized in breast cancer, AT-derived estrogen may also play a role in other cancers. For example, the development of endometrial cancer is associated with obesity, and blockade of estrogen signaling through the administration of synthetic progestogens is employed as a mode of therapy in type 1 endometrial cancer patient subsets [102, 103]. The control of ER-mediated genomic signaling in endometrial tissue varies from the breast, however, the pathways activated remain similar and also have a pro-oncogenic effect if deregulated [104]. However, endometrial cancer may differ from breast cancer in that ER signaling appears most important in early-stage disease where it is involved in carcinogenesis but may not be involved in disease progression due to reported loss in ER expression documented in metastatic endometrial cancer [105]. This is reflected in the literature, as epidemiological studies report a clear association between obesity and endometrial cancer risk, but mixed results with respect to the association between obesity and endometrial cancer outcomes [106]. This may be in part due to the lower incidence rate of this cancer. However, it may also be explained by a phenomenon termed the "obesity paradox", wherein an increased BMI is associated with better survival outcomes in patients with certain cancer types (discussed in Section 3 below).

2.4.2 Androgen signaling

Androgens are the family of steroid hormones that regulate the development of male sex characteristics, the predominant of which is testosterone which signals via the androgen receptor (AR) once converted to its active metabolite dihydrotestosterone (DHT). The link between the AT and androgen signaling is not as well characterized as that of estrogen but it is known that excess adiposity can disrupt signaling along this axis. Unlike other cancer types described by the IARC working group, obesity is not a risk factor for the development of prostate cancer, however, it is reported to impact outcome in these patients suggesting that AT-derived factors influence its growth and progression [107, 108]. The prostate is surrounded by its own AT depot (peri-prostatic AT) which likely impacts prostate cancer within the local environment in addition to the systemic effect of obesity/AT dysfunction. Excess adiposity impacts androgen biosynthesis in a sex-specific manner with androgen levels overall decreased in men with obesity [109, 110]. In the context of prostate cancer, this may appear counterintuitive given the dependence of prostate cancer growth on androgen signaling, however, many studies have shown prostate cancer cells to inhibit proliferation in response to androgen exposure [111, 112]. Considering this, it is likely that the pro-tumor influence of the AT on prostate cancer is attributed to other AT-derived factors which may activate aberrant AR signaling in an alternative manner.

Inflammatory cytokines such as IL-6 and IL-8, often associated with obesity-associated AT dysfunction, have been shown to activate the AR in a ligand-independent manner putatively linking the AT to poor prostate cancer outcomes in this context [113]. IL-6 in particular has been identified as a prognostic factor in prostate cancer, and elevated serum IL-6 is correlated with the clinical stage of the disease and reduced survival [114]. The resulting downstream effects of alternative AR activation in prostate cancer appear variable depending on AR status and/or context of exposure to these signals. IL-6, for example, is reported to activate STAT3 and MAPK (mitogen-activated protein kinase) signaling in the androgen-sensitive AR single mutant LNCap cell line [115], however, only MAPK activation is seen in AR wild-type LAPC-4 and AR double mutant MDA PCA 2b cells [116, 117]. Additionally, MDA PCA 2b cells adopt an enhanced proliferative phenotype in response to chronic IL-6 exposure [117]. Some studies have shown no effect or inhibition of proliferation on LNCap cells in response to IL-6 exposure which is supported by other studies demonstrating that IL-6-mediated enhanced activation of AR signaling requires the presence of androgens for its activation and expression of AR target genes [118, 119]. This observed synergy may pose as a mechanism to reduce the threshold for AR activation in the absence of androgens. However, there have also been reports of IL-6-regulated activation of androgen response element (ARE)-mediated gene activation in prostate cancer cell lines when treated in the absence of androgen [116]. Similarly, IL-8 has been shown to positively regulate proliferation in prostate cancer cell lines while also upregulating AR-regulated genes implicating this cytokine in the ligand-independent activation of AR in a similar manner to IL-6 [120]. Alternative activation of the AR via these mechanisms is thought to be of particular importance in castration-resistant prostate cancer, where cells are no longer dependent on androgens for growth and employ alternative mechanisms for survival. Although clinical studies have identified these cytokines as key players in prostate cancer, evidence directly linking AT-derived inflammatory cytokines to these observations is somewhat lacking and requires further investigation.

2.4.3 Adipokines

Adipokines encompass an array of bioactive molecules secreted by adipocytes which have a range of physiological functions, including maintaining glucose and energy homeostasis, appetite, and inflammation. Of these, leptin and adiponectin are two of the best characterized, both for their normal physiological roles and their roles in promoting obesity-associated pro-tumorigenic activity. Under normal physiological conditions, a strict adiponectin/leptin ratio is maintained. Functionally, leptin serves to promote cellular proliferation and inflammation, while adiponectin has pro-apoptotic and anti-inflammatory effects. However, the adiponectin/leptin ratio can become altered in people with obesity and may have clinical potential in predicting the onset of obesity-associated diseases in metabolically unhealthy lean individuals [121, 122].

Under normal physiological conditions, leptin is an anti-apoptotic and pro-inflammatory molecule, with additional functions in angiogenesis, modulating glucose and insulin homeostasis, and suppressing appetite [123–125]. Secretion of leptin is directly regulated by the mass of an individual and is increased in people with obesity, which can result in leptin resistance [126, 127].

Upon binding of leptin to its receptor (ObR), several intracellular pathways are activated, such as the extracellular signal-regulated kinase 1/2 (ERK1/2), Janus kinase (JAK)/STAT, and MAPK/phosphoinositide 3-kinase (PI3K) pathways. Many of the activated pathways have been implicated in cancer, and can affect cell capabilities such as growth and survival, proliferation, migration, invasion, and inflammation to promote cell transformation and tumor progression [128]. These effects are thought to be primarily mediated through the MAPK pathways.

Leptin potentiates proliferative signaling in a variety of cancer models including breast, ovarian, endometrial, and prostate by modulating cell cycle progression/regulatory genes such as proliferating cell nuclear antigen (PCNA), p21, and Cyclin-D1, while also inhibiting pro-apoptotic gene expression [129–131]. Furthermore, leptin has also been shown to bind the ERα receptor in ovarian, endometrial, and breast cancer cells, thus stimulating cancer cell proliferation [132]. Leptin treatment of cancer cell lines enhances their invasion and migratory profiles [133, 134]. In particular, leptin promotes the secretion of matrix metalloproteinase (MMP) enzymes, which degrade the extracellular matrix (ECM) and promote matrix remodeling of the stroma to facilitate cancer cell migration [135, 136]. Leptin also stimulates transcription of the vascular endothelial growth factor (VEGF) gene, promoting angiogenesis to allow oxygen to reach expanding cells, which may be hijacked by incipient tumors to favor their survival [137]. Furthermore, increased serum cancer stem cell numbers correlated with increased leptin levels in breast cancer, demonstrating that it can also promote stemness [138]. In pancreatic cancer, leptin has been shown to promote expression of the cancer stem cell markers CD24, CD44, and ESA [139].

The use of leptin as clinical biomarker has not been validated and correlations of expression with disease risk and outcome have yielded mixed results [140–143]. However, some studies have shown that elevated serum leptin levels are indicative of breast cancer risk irrespective of BMI indicating a direct link to cancer independent of obesity [144].

Adiponectin is a pro-apoptotic and anti-inflammatory adipokine under normal physiological conditions and its secretion has been reported to decrease with increasing adiposity [145, 146]. In contrast to many other adipokines, lower circulating levels of adiponectin are associated with increased risk of cancers such as breast, ovarian, and prostate [147–154]. For example, lower serum levels of adiponectin have been associated with increased breast cancer risk and higher-grade tumors [154]. In breast cancer cells, exogenous adiponectin impaired stem cell renewal, in direct contrast to leptin [138]. Furthermore, *in vivo* administration of adiponectin results in decreased tumor growth, proliferation, invasion, and migration, further suggesting that its reduced secretion may favor tumor growth [155–159].

Expression of adiponectin receptors (AdipoR1 and AdipoR2) in cancer cells has been reported, indicating that adiponectin can act directly on cancer cells [158, 160]. Interestingly, cancers associated with obesity were significantly more likely to express adiponectin receptors, further implicating adiponectin signaling in obesity-associated carcinogenesis [161]. Upon binding of adiponectin to its cell surface receptors, the AMP-activated protein kinase (AMPK) pathway is activated, while the Wnt/β-catenin, ERK1/2, NADPH oxidase, STAT3, and NF-κB pathways are all inhibited. The AMPK pathway is the most commonly implicated pathway in the link between adiponectin signaling and cancer. When activated, it induces expression of cell cycle regulators p53, p27, and p21, resulting in cell cycle arrest [162]. Exogenous treatment of breast and ovarian cancer cell lines with adiponectin resulted in downregulation of cell cycle proteins such as cyclin D1, preventing cells from entering S and G2/M phases of the cell cycle [163, 164]. In addition to inducing cell cycle arrest, adiponectin can promote apoptosis in several cancer cell lines via the upregulation of Bax, downregulation of Bcl-2, and activation of caspases 3, 8, and 9 [165–168]. Therefore, reduced adiponectin production by dysfunctional AT and the resultant decrease in AMPK signaling may impair cell cycle arrest and apoptotic cell death mechanisms in cancer cells.

Adiponectin has also been shown to regulate the functions of growth factors such as platelet-derived growth factor-BB (PDGF-BB), basic fibroblast growth factor (bFGF), and heparin-binding EGF-like growth factor (HB-EGF). Binding and sequestering of these growth factors by adiponectin may reduce their bioavailability to cells, thus impairing DNA synthesis, cell proliferation, and migration, as demonstrated in smooth muscle cells [169, 170]. Thus, it is likely that increased bioavailability of these growth factors as a consequence of obesity-associated adiponectin depletion may promote tumorigenic pathways. Indeed, increased growth factor signaling is well recognized for enabling sustained proliferation in cancer cells [41, 42].

2.5 The role of AT-induced oxidative stress in cancer

Individuals with obesity display oxidative stress systemically and locally within the AT which exacerbates AT dysfunction and can contribute to a number of diseases such as cancer. Oxidative stress describes the imbalance between pro- and antioxidant species within the body and is often characterized by an accumulation of pro-oxidants such as reactive oxygen species (ROS) and free radicals. These molecules are potent signaling effectors that are required under normal physiological conditions but imbalances in their levels can significantly alter other intracellular signaling pathways and cause severe disruption to normal cellular function. Obesity-associated AT dysfunction is linked to an increase in oxidative stress and it is postulated that this can occur even in the early stages of obesity, implicating it in the development of obesity but also as a consequence of obesity [171]. Lipid peroxidation, which is a common consequence of the presence of excess oxidative species, has been positively correlated with BMI in human subjects and those with obesity have significantly higher circulating markers of oxidative stress than their lean counterparts [172, 173]. AT expression of enzymes involved in the production of ROS, such as nicotinamide adenine dinucleotide phosphate (NADPH) oxidase, is also increased in models of obesity while deletion of the NOX4 gene prevents the onset of obesity-induced insulin resistance and inflammation directly implicating the AT in the process of oxidative stress [172, 174]. The production of ROS is intimately linked with the innate immune response and it is likely that AT-resident immune cells are responsible by in large for obesity-linked oxidative stress. Macrophages contribute to a large proportion of ROS production within the body and upon activation go through a respiratory burst where they produce large amounts of ROS via the NADPH oxidase enzyme. Inhibition of macrophage proliferation in vivo is effective in attenuating obesity-induced oxidative stress within the AT [175]. It is now widely accepted that ROS production by macrophages is essential to their ability to mount an immune response to invading pathogens via the induction of immune regulatory pathways such as NF-κB and JAK/STAT signaling. However, within dysfunctional AT, this response is constitutively activated resulting in local tissue damage.

Prolonged oxidative stress is considered to be directly implicated in carcinogenesis due to the ability of ROS to alter cell signaling pathways and induce DNA damage. DNA bases are highly susceptible to oxidation, resulting in base alterations and consequent genetic mutations that may affect oncogenes and/or tumor suppressor genes. ROS are also capable of inducing both double and single-strand DNA breaks in addition to DNA cross-linking all of which increase the likelihood of errors in DNA repair when they occur persistently. Cellular processes linked to carcinogenesis such as proliferation, apoptosis, and adhesion can also be affected by oxidative stress due to changes in gene expression. The presence of hydrogen peroxide (H_2O_2) has been shown to activate signaling pathways related to tumorigenesis such as NF-κB and MAPK pathways [176]. Although the exact mechanisms involving ROS in the induction of these signaling cascades are not fully understood, studies have shown that anti-oxidants can block the activation of NF-κB signaling induced by multiple different stimuli [177–179]. Although, this has been mostly associated with transient or low-level exposure to ROS which may be associated with earlier stages of AT dysfunction as opposed to that observed in later stages of obesity. Studies have shown ROS to be involved in pro-tumorigenic processes not only in cancer initiation but also in cancer progression. ROS has been directly implicated in promoting a migratory phenotype in bladder cancer cell lines via the ROS-dependent activation of Hypoxia-inducible factor (HIF) to upregulate MMP-1 expression [180]. Contrastingly, NADPH oxidase inhibitors can prevent ROS-induced invasion and migration by suppressing ERK1/2 MAPK signaling [181]. ROS is also a known inducer of angiogenesis and has been linked to neo-angiogenesis via the upregulation of HIF-1α and VEGF transcriptional mechanisms in ovarian cancer cells [182].

2.6 Cancer-associated adipocytes (CAAs)

Communication between the various cell populations within the TME is imperative for the growth and metastatic spread of all tumors. As we now know, communication between tumor-adjacent adipocytes and cancer cells is bidirectional and cancer cells are capable of altering adipocyte phenotype in order to support their growth and survival. These adipocyte populations have distinct characteristics compared to normal mature AT-resident adipocytes and were formally characterized by Dirat and colleagues over a decade ago [183]. These adipocytes, termed cancer-associated adipocytes (CAAs), display an activated phenotype and exhibit reprogramming of their metabolic and inflammatory profiles. Direct cancer cell contact induces a de-differentiated state in CAAs which adopt a more mesenchymal-like morphology, appearing similar to fibroblast populations [184]. Furthermore, this contact causes a reduction in expression of terminal differentiation markers normally expressed by mature adipocytes such as hormone-sensitive lipase (HSL), resistin, and adiponectin [183]. This de-differentiation process is suggested to be mediated by cancer-secreted factors which unsurprisingly disrupt pathways involved in cell fate determination and cell survival such as Wnt/β-catenin and Hippo signaling pathways. Cancer cells secrete both Wnt3 and Wnt5a in response to adipocyte-derived inflammatory signals, which can activate Wnt/β-catenin signaling to reduce adipocyte differentiation marker expression [184, 185]. Other pathways suggested to be involved include the Hippo signaling pathway which is activated upon co-culture of mature adipocytes with breast cancer cells [186]. *In vivo* administration of verteporfin (Yes-associated protein/transcriptional coactivator PDZ-binding motif or YAP/TAZ inhibitor) in diet-induced obesity tumor models both restores a differentiated adipocyte phenotype and inhibits tumor progression [186]. CAAs are highly metabolically active cells and upregulate lipolysis in order to provide additional FFAs for cancer cell uptake and utilization and are therefore also characterized by a decrease in intracellular lipid content [187]. These cells are primed to express and secrete various factors including inflammatory cytokines, chemokines, adipokines, growth/angiogenic factors, and matrix remodeling enzymes in response to cancer cell contact as described within the previous sections of this chapter.

3. Lifestyle interventions in obesity-associated cancers

Obesity-associated carcinogenesis is intrinsically linked to the dysregulated signaling pathways, increased inflammation, and altered secretome associated with dysfunctional AT. In addition to epidemiological evidence showing an association between obesity and cancer incidence, obesity has been associated with cancer recurrence and poorer survival outcomes in cancers such as endometrial, breast, and colon [188–190]. Moreover, some patients with cancer and obesity experience an increase in treatment-related adverse events. For example, in patients with cervical cancer, greater radiation treatment-induced toxicity has been reported compared to leaner patients [191]. In one study, patients with breast cancer and obesity receiving sentinel lymph node dissection had a greater risk of developing lymphedema, a well-known postoperative complication of this procedure, compared to leaner patients [192].

Given the multitude of pathways and mechanisms linking AT and carcinogenesis, targeted therapeutic approaches are difficult to devise. Therefore, logical therapeutic strategies for obesity-associated cancers might include those that target the tumor while also targeting obesity to restore AT functionality. Lifestyle interventions that promote healthy behaviors, such as changes to diet and increased physical activity, may therefore improve treatment responses and mortality. In 2018, the World Cancer Research Fund (WCRF)/American Institute for Cancer Research (AICR) published

Cancer Prevention Recommendations, a set of guidelines that encourage healthy lifestyle behaviors to reduce cancer risk and include recommendations on diet, physical activity, maintenance of healthy body weight, and alcohol consumption [193]. A systematic review from 2023 found that greater adherence to these guidelines was associated with a reduced risk of developing breast, colorectal, and lung cancers, although this association was not found for prostate cancer [194].

Mechanistically, weight loss in humans has been shown to result in increased adiponectin expression and secretion, while leptin levels are decreased [195–201]. Furthermore, several studies have shown that weight loss is associated with a decrease in markers of inflammation such as TNFα, C-reactive protein (CRP), as well as a decrease in serum insulin, estrogen, and testosterone levels [197, 201–205]. However, another study suggested that even after weight loss, tissue-resident macrophages sustain AT inflammation in formerly obese mice [206]. In humans with obesity who lost weight following bariatric surgery, decreased CLS formation, decreased insulin resistance, and decreased circulating levels of pro-inflammatory mediators were observed [56]. Interestingly, rapid weight loss resulting from a very low-calorie diet caused increased density of CLS in subcutaneous AT; however, this was associated with a decrease in systemic biomarkers of inflammation and insulin resistance and was not associated with increased expression of pro-inflammatory genes [207]. Furthermore, one study demonstrated that in women with obesity placed on a very low-calorie diet, expression of pro inflammatory markers in subcutaneous AT was unchanged in the early phases, but increased in the later phases of the diet [208]. In addition, physical activity in humans has been shown to trigger IL-6 production from muscle fibers, which can stimulate the production of the anti-inflammatory cytokines IL-1Ra and IL-10 [209, 210]. In mice, IL-6 can also activate AMPK signaling and inhibit TNFα production [211–214]. Additionally, high-intensity exercise in mice promoted macrophage polarization to anti-inflammatory phenotypes [215]. It has also been shown that, lipopolysaccharide-induced inflammation could be attenuated in physically active mice compared to sedentary controls [216]. Therefore, it could be theorized that weight loss and physical activity may help to reverse obesity-associated AT phenotypes that have been implicated in supporting tumor growth.

Studies investigating the effects of such lifestyle interventions have produced mixed results. Some studies in patients with breast and colon cancers suggest that increased levels of physical activity are associated with a reduced mortality risk [196–198]. Furthermore, one systematic review found an association between increased physical activity and a larger reduction in relative risk for bladder, colon, breast, and esophageal cancers when compared to lower levels of physical activity [217]. However, evidence of such an effect was limited in ovarian, pancreatic, and prostate cancer. Another study found that dietary weight loss, alone or in combination with exercise, significantly improved IR, in postmenopausal women with overweight or obesity, which was not observed with exercise alone [218]. A study investigating the effects of recent weight loss on cancer risk in health workers found a significantly increased risk of cancer development in those who experienced recent weight loss of more than 10% of their body weight compared to those who had not lost weight over the same period [219]. Of note, individuals who intentionally lost weight by adopting weight-loss-promoting behaviors had a decreased risk of cancer compared to those who unintentionally lost weight. Furthermore, one systematic review which looked at weight loss and cancer incidence using 34 studies found a significant reduction in cancer incidence in individuals who lost weight in 16 of the studies but observed no such relationship in the remaining 18 studies [220].

Despite some evidence demonstrating the benefits of lifestyle interventions in reducing cancer incidence and improving treatment and survival outcomes, these benefits may be specific to cancer type. Several studies have been published suggesting that increased BMI is associated with better cancer treatment outcomes and decreased mortality in patients with a higher BMI compared to a lower BMI in esophageal, prostate, renal, gastric cervical, breast, lymphoma leukemia, colorectal, and lung cancers [221–230]. This phenomenon suggesting a positive correlation between obesity/increased BMI and treatment response or survival outcome has been termed the "obesity paradox". The mechanisms underlying this phenomenon are not fully understood, but evidence is mounting to suggest that functional AT in obesity may serve protective functions. For example, patients with advanced cancer commonly experience cachexia, a disorder characterized by wasting of AT and skeletal muscle, resulting in weight loss, and this is a well-established risk factor for cancer mortality [231]. Excess AT in obesity may serve as a reserve for energy and nutrients, favoring outcomes of cancer treatment in these patients [222]. Additionally, study limitations including confounding factors, reverse causation, and the use of BMI as a proxy for obesity are thought to partially explain it [232–234].

A systematic review conducted by Ligibel et al. aimed to provide guidance relating to physical activity, diet, and weight management for adults undergoing cancer treatment. The authors concluded that current evidence is insufficient to enable clinical guidelines on intentional weight loss or weight management for patients actively undergoing cancer treatment to be provided [235]. These conflicting and seemingly cancer-type-dependent associations and outcomes indicate that further studies are needed to conclusively determine the effects of adiposity on cancer survivorship and treatment response before lifestyle interventions are implemented.

4. Conclusions

The biological mechanisms underlying AT dysfunction and its contribution to cancer are complex, involving crosstalk between several cell types within both the AT microenvironment and the TME, multiple signaling pathways, and both local and systemic elements. Although fully encompassing the AT-cancer landscape within this chapter is not possible, we have focused on the mechanisms that have been best characterized to date, which are summarized below in **Figure 1**.

The alarming increase in obesity rates over recent decades has driven research into the functional attributes of adipocytes in this context, particularly due to the association of obesity with several secondary conditions. Dysfunctional adipocytes, characteristically described in obesity, are now understood to be a primary etiological agent. Most recently, epidemiological findings have linked several cancer types to obesity, although the underlying mechanisms which explain this association remain to be fully elucidated. In isolation, cancer itself is well characterized as a multifactorial process dependent on cells and nutrients within the TME to survive, challenging the archaic idea of cancer cells alone driving disease progression. The emerging picture of the AT is similar, where the local AT microenvironment and cell-cell crosstalk dictate disease pathogenesis. The impact of AT dysfunction on cancer growth is documented on both systemic and local levels, as both circulating factors and direct interaction between cancer cells and adjacent tissues including AT are imperative for the growth and progression of the disease. AT cells known to display a tumor-associated phenotype in obesity-associated AT dysfunction and interact with cancer cells include immune

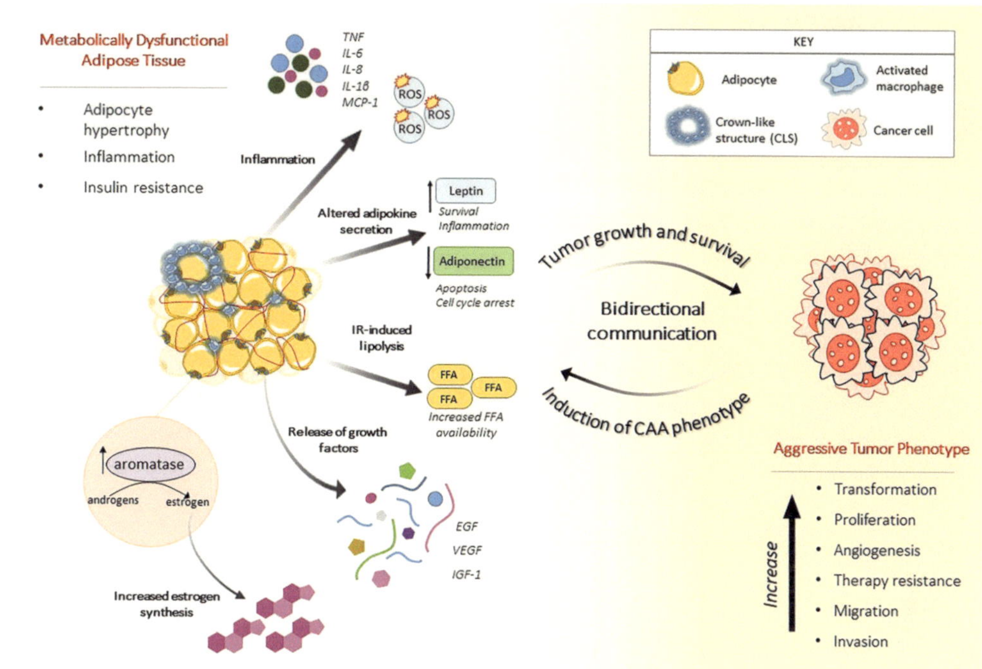

Figure 1.
Adipose tissue (AT) and cancer cell bidirectional communication supports tumor growth and progression. Disturbances in AT homeostasis are observed in conditions such as obesity resulting in increased free fatty acid (FFA) release, inflammation, and subsequent insulin resistance (IR) within the AT rendering it metabolically and immunologically dysfunctional. Factors secreted from the AT (cytokines, chemokines, adipokines, FFAs, growth factors, and estrogen) can promote an aggressive tumor phenotype by supporting processes involved in cancer initiation, growth, and metastasis. Simultaneously, cancer cells can induce a cancer-associated adipocyte (CAA) phenotype in adjacent adipocytes, conditioning them to produce factors to further support pro-tumorigenic activities within the TME.

cells, stromal cells, endothelial cells, and adipocytes themselves. Crosstalk between these cells can induce physiological changes to tumor growth including, but not limited to, DNA damage repair, cell growth and survival, differentiation, angiogenesis, and inflammatory responses. As with AT, the biology of the TME is significantly altered in metabolically dysfunctional states, and this can be due to the influence of the AT itself.

Taken together, there exists an intimate and intricate relationship between dysfunctional AT and the TME in the context of obesity, which warrants further investigation. In particular, this relationship should be a factor of consideration in cancer therapeutics and treatment regimes. Obesity is a well-established risk factor for 13 cancer types, as described by the IARC working group, and also influences cancer outcomes for several other cancer types. Therefore, there is a premise to consider patients with cancer and obesity as a separate subset of patients in terms of prognosis and disease management. Novel therapeutic strategies should consider the impact of the AT and potentially aim to reduce the physiological burden of obesity-associated metabolic deregulation while also targeting the AT-induced molecular changes within the tumor and the TME. However, further work in identifying and characterizing patient subsets that will benefit most from these types of interventions is required before novel therapeutic strategies can be developed and employed for the treatment of obesity-associated cancer.

Acknowledgements

This work was funded by Research Ireland.

Author details

Noor Bakour*, Claudine Duggan and Stephanie L. Annett
School of Pharmacy and Biomolecular Sciences, RCSI University of Medicine and Health Sciences, Dublin, Ireland

*Address all correspondence to: noorbakour20@rcsi.ie

IntechOpen

© 2025 The Author(s). Licensee IntechOpen. This chapter is distributed under the terms of the Creative Commons Attribution License (http://creativecommons.org/licenses/by/3.0), which permits unrestricted use, distribution, and reproduction in any medium, provided the original work is properly cited.

References

[1] Fryar CDCM, Afful J. Prevalence of Overweight, Obesity, and Severe Obesity among Adults Aged 20 and Over: United States, 1960-1962 through 2017-2018. NCHS Health E-Statistics; 2020. Available from: https://www.cdc.gov/nchs/data/hestat/obesity-adult-17-18/obesity-adult.htm

[2] Cooper C, Backholder K, Bell C, Cameron AJ, Jacons J, Patrick R, et al. WHO European Regional Obesity Report 2022. Copenhagen: WHO Regional Office for Europe; 2022. Available from: https://www.who.int/europe/publications/i/item/9789289057738

[3] Sung H, Siegel RL, Torre LA, Pearson-Stuttard J, Islami F, Fedewa SA, et al. Global patterns in excess body weight and the associated cancer burden. CA: A Cancer Journal for Clinicians. 2019;**69**(2):88-112

[4] Bray F, Laversanne M, Sung H, Ferlay J, Siegal RL, Soerjomataram I, Jemal A. World Health Organization: Global Cancer Observatory (GLOBOCAN). 2022. Available from: https://gco.iarc.fr/en

[5] Ferlay JEM, Lam F, Colombet M, Mery L, Piñeros M, et al. Global Cancer Observatory: Cancer Today. Lyon: International Agency for Research on Cancer; 2020 Available from: https://gco.iarc.fr/today/en

[6] Setiawan VW, Yang HP, Pike MC, McCann SE, Yu H, Xiang YB, et al. Type I and II endometrial cancers: Have they different risk factors? Journal of Clinical Oncology. 2013;**31**(20):2607-2618

[7] Hoyo C, Cook MB, Kamangar F, Freedman ND, Whiteman DC, Bernstein L, et al. Body mass index in relation to oesophageal and oesophagogastric junction adenocarcinomas: A pooled analysis from the international BEACON consortium. International Journal of Epidemiology. 2012;**41**(6):1706-1718

[8] Wang F, Xu Y. Body mass index and risk of renal cell cancer: A dose-response meta-analysis of published cohort studies. International Journal of Cancer. 2014;**135**(7):1673-1686

[9] Chen Y, Liu L, Wang X, Wang J, Yan Z, Cheng J, et al. Body mass index and risk of gastric cancer: A meta-analysis of a population with more than ten million from 24 prospective studies. Cancer Epidemiology, Biomarkers and Prevention. 2013;**22**(8):1395-1408

[10] Chen Y, Wang X, Wang J, Yan Z, Luo J. Excess body weight and the risk of primary liver cancer: An updated meta-analysis of prospective studies. European Journal of Cancer. 2012;**48**(14):2137-2145

[11] Li L, Gan Y, Li W, Wu C, Lu Z. Overweight, obesity and the risk of gallbladder and extrahepatic bile duct cancers: A meta-analysis of observational studies. Obesity (Silver Spring). 2016;**24**(8):1786-1802

[12] Niedermaier T, Behrens G, Schmid D, Schlecht I, Fischer B, Leitzmann MF. Body mass index, physical activity, and risk of adult meningioma and glioma: A meta-analysis. Neurology. 2015;**85**(15):1342-1350

[13] Genkinger JM, Spiegelman D, Anderson KE, Bernstein L, van den Brandt PA, Calle EE, et al. A pooled analysis of 14 cohort studies of anthropometric factors and pancreatic

cancer risk. International Journal of Cancer. 2011;**129**(7):1708-1717

[14] Teras LR, Kitahara CM, Birmann BM, Hartge PA, Wang SS, Robien K, et al. Body size and multiple myeloma mortality: A pooled analysis of 20 prospective studies. British Journal of Haematology. 2014;**166**(5):667-676

[15] Ma Y, Yang Y, Wang F, Zhang P, Shi C, Zou Y, et al. Obesity and risk of colorectal cancer: A systematic review of prospective studies. PLoS One. 2013;**8**(1):e53916

[16] Renehan AG, Tyson M, Egger M, Heller RF, Zwahlen M. Body-mass index and incidence of cancer: A systematic review and meta-analysis of prospective observational studies. Lancet. 2008;**371**(9612):569-578

[17] Ovarian cancer and body size. Individual participant meta-analysis including 25,157 women with ovarian cancer from 47 epidemiological studies. PLoS Medicine. 2012;**9**(4):e1001200

[18] Kitahara CM, McCullough ML, Franceschi S, Rinaldi S, Wolk A, Neta G, et al. Anthropometric factors and thyroid Cancer risk by histological subtype: Pooled analysis of 22 prospective studies. Thyroid. 2016;**26**(2):306-318

[19] Lauby-Secretan B, Scoccianti C, Loomis D, Grosse Y, Bianchini F, Straif K. Body fatness and cancer--Viewpoint of the IARC working group. The New England Journal of Medicine. 2016;**375**(8):794-798

[20] Zhi X, Kuang XH, Liu K, Li J. The global burden and temporal trend of cancer attributable to high body mass index: Estimates from the global burden of disease study 2019. Frontiers in Nutrition. 2022;**9**:918330

[21] Tan DJH, Ng CH, Muthiah M, Yong JN, Chee D, Teng M, et al. Rising global burden of cancer attributable to high BMI from 2010 to 2019. Metabolism. 2024;**152**:155744

[22] Pearson-Stuttard J, Zhou B, Kontis V, Bentham J, Gunter MJ, Ezzati M. Worldwide burden of cancer attributable to diabetes and high body-mass index: A comparative risk assessment. The Lancet Diabetes and Endocrinology. 2018;**6**(6):e6-e15

[23] Lee H. Obesity-associated cancers: Evidence from studies in mouse models. Cells. 2022;**11**(9)

[24] Duan P, Hu C, Quan C, Yi X, Zhou W, Yuan M, et al. Body mass index and risk of lung cancer: Systematic review and dose-response meta-analysis. Scientific Reports. 2015;**5**:16938

[25] Choi YJ, Lee DH, Han K, Yoon H, Shin CM, Park YS, et al. Joint effects of low body mass index and alcohol consumption on developing esophageal squamous cell cancer: A Korean nationwide population-based cohort study. Asian Pacific Journal of Cancer Prevention. 2017;**18**(7):1881-1887

[26] Emont MP, Jacobs C, Essene AL, Pant D, Tenen D, Colleluori G, et al. A single-cell atlas of human and mouse white adipose tissue. Nature. 2022;**603**(7903):926-933

[27] Salmon H, Franciszkiewicz K, Damotte D, Dieu-Nosjean MC, Validire P, Trautmann A, et al. Matrix architecture defines the preferential localization and migration of T cells into the stroma of human lung tumors. The Journal of Clinical Investigation. 2012;**122**(3):899-910

[28] Arner P, Bernard S, Salehpour M, Possnert G, Liebl J, Steier P, et al.

Dynamics of human adipose lipid turnover in health and metabolic disease. Nature. 2011;**478**(7367):110-113

[29] Hartwig S, De Filippo E, Goddeke S, Knebel B, Kotzka J, Al-Hasani H, et al. Exosomal proteins constitute an essential part of the human adipose tissue secretome. Biochimica et Biophysica Acta (BBA) - Proteins and Proteomics. 2019;**1867**(12):140172

[30] Gastaldelli A, Gaggini M, DeFronzo RA. Role of adipose tissue insulin resistance in the natural history of type 2 diabetes: Results from the San Antonio metabolism study. Diabetes. 2017;**66**(4):815-822

[31] Cao Y. Adipose tissue angiogenesis as a therapeutic target for obesity and metabolic diseases. Nature Reviews. Drug Discovery. 2010;**9**(2):107-115

[32] Cao Y. Angiogenesis modulates adipogenesis and obesity. The Journal of Clinical Investigation. 2007;**117**(9):2362-2368

[33] Cartwright MJ, Tchkonia T, Kirkland JL. Aging in adipocytes: Potential impact of inherent, depot-specific mechanisms. Experimental Gerontology. 2007;**42**(6):463-471

[34] Spalding KL, Arner E, Westermark PO, Bernard S, Buchholz BA, Bergmann O, et al. Dynamics of fat cell turnover in humans. Nature. 2008;**453**(7196):783-787

[35] Heinonen S, Buzkova J, Muniandy M, Kaksonen R, Ollikainen M, Ismail K, et al. Impaired mitochondrial biogenesis in adipose tissue in acquired obesity. Diabetes. 2015;**64**(9):3135-3145

[36] Sorisky A, Magun R, Gagnon AM. Adipose cell apoptosis: Death in the energy depot. International Journal of Obesity and Related Metabolic Disorders. 2000;**24**(Suppl. 4):S3-S7

[37] Strissel KJ, Stancheva Z, Miyoshi H, Perfield JW 2nd, DeFuria J, Jick Z, et al. Adipocyte death, adipose tissue remodeling, and obesity complications. Diabetes. 2007;**56**(12):2910-2918

[38] Trayhurn P. Hypoxia and adipose tissue function and dysfunction in obesity. Physiological Reviews. 2013;**93**(1):1-21

[39] Trim WV, Lynch L. Immune and non-immune functions of adipose tissue leukocytes. Nature Reviews. Immunology. 2022;**22**(6):371-386

[40] Grant RW, Dixit VD. Adipose tissue as an immunological organ. Obesity (Silver Spring). 2015;**23**(3):512-518

[41] Hanahan D, Weinberg RA. The hallmarks of cancer. Cell. 2000;**100**(1):57-70

[42] Hanahan D, Weinberg RA. Hallmarks of cancer: The next generation. Cell. 2011;**144**(5):646-674

[43] Fest J, Ruiter R, Mulder M, Groot Koerkamp B, Ikram MA, Stricker BH, et al. The systemic immune-inflammation index is associated with an increased risk of incident cancer-a population-based cohort study. International Journal of Cancer. 2020;**146**(3):692-698

[44] Nost TH, Alcala K, Urbarova I, Byrne KS, Guida F, Sandanger TM, et al. Systemic inflammation markers and cancer incidence in the UK biobank. European Journal of Epidemiology. 2021;**36**(8):841-848

[45] Volkova E, Willis JA, Wells JE, Robinson BA, Dachs GU, Currie MJ. Association of angiopoietin-2, C-reactive protein and markers of obesity and

insulin resistance with survival outcome in colorectal cancer. British Journal of Cancer. 2011;**104**(1):51-59

[46] Xu H, Barnes GT, Yang Q, Tan G, Yang D, Chou CJ, et al. Chronic inflammation in fat plays a crucial role in the development of obesity-related insulin resistance. The Journal of Clinical Investigation. 2003;**112**(12):1821-1830

[47] Martinez O, de Victoria E, Xu X, Koska J, Francisco AM, Scalise M, et al. Macrophage content in subcutaneous adipose tissue: Associations with adiposity, age, inflammatory markers, and whole-body insulin action in healthy Pima Indians. Diabetes. 2009;**58**(2):385-393

[48] Osborn O, Olefsky JM. The cellular and signaling networks linking the immune system and metabolism in disease. Nature Medicine. 2012;**18**(3):363-374

[49] Weisberg SP, McCann D, Desai M, Rosenbaum M, Leibel RL, Ferrante AW Jr. Obesity is associated with macrophage accumulation in adipose tissue. The Journal of Clinical Investigation. 2003;**112**(12):1796-1808

[50] Deiuliis J, Shah Z, Shah N, Needleman B, Mikami D, Narula V, et al. Visceral adipose inflammation in obesity is associated with critical alterations in tregulatory cell numbers. PLoS One. 2011;**6**(1):e16376

[51] Deng T, Lyon CJ, Bergin S, Caligiuri MA, Hsueh WA. Obesity, inflammation, and cancer. Annual Review of Pathology. 2016;**11**:421-449

[52] Nishimura S, Manabe I, Nagasaki M, Eto K, Yamashita H, Ohsugi M, et al. CD8+ effector T cells contribute to macrophage recruitment and adipose tissue inflammation in obesity. Nature Medicine. 2009;**15**(8):914-920

[53] van der Weerd K, Dik WA, Schrijver B, Schweitzer DH, Langerak AW, Drexhage HA, et al. Morbidly obese human subjects have increased peripheral blood CD4+ T cells with skewing toward a Treg- and Th2-dominated phenotype. Diabetes. 2012;**61**(2):401-408

[54] Zeyda M, Huber J, Prager G, Stulnig TM. Inflammation correlates with markers of T-cell subsets including regulatory T cells in adipose tissue from obese patients. Obesity (Silver Spring). 2011;**19**(4):743-748

[55] Lumeng CN, Bodzin JL, Saltiel AR. Obesity induces a phenotypic switch in adipose tissue macrophage polarization. The Journal of Clinical Investigation. 2007;**117**(1):175-184

[56] Cancello R, Henegar C, Viguerie N, Taleb S, Poitou C, Rouault C, et al. Reduction of macrophage infiltration and chemoattractant gene expression changes in white adipose tissue of morbidly obese subjects after surgery-induced weight loss. Diabetes. 2005;**54**(8):2277-2286

[57] Cinti S, Mitchell G, Barbatelli G, Murano I, Ceresi E, Faloia E, et al. Adipocyte death defines macrophage localization and function in adipose tissue of obese mice and humans. Journal of Lipid Research. 2005;**46**(11):2347-2355

[58] Murano I, Barbatelli G, Parisani V, Latini C, Muzzonigro G, Castellucci M, et al. Dead adipocytes, detected as crown-like structures, are prevalent in visceral fat depots of genetically obese mice. Journal of Lipid Research. 2008;**49**(7):1562-1568

[59] Shi H, Kokoeva MV, Inouye K, Tzameli I, Yin H, Flier JS. TLR4 links innate immunity and fatty acid-induced insulin resistance. The Journal of Clinical Investigation. 2006;**116**(11):3015-3025

[60] Shapiro H, Pecht T, Shaco-Levy R, Harman-Boehm I, Kirshtein B, Kuperman Y, et al. Adipose tissue foam cells are present in human obesity. The Journal of Clinical Endocrinology and Metabolism. 2013;**98**(3):1173-1181

[61] Nicklas BJ, Rogus EM, Colman EG, Goldberg AP. Visceral adiposity, increased adipocyte lipolysis, and metabolic dysfunction in obese postmenopausal women. The American Journal of Physiology. 1996;**270**(1 Pt 1):E72-E78

[62] Lee JY, Ye J, Gao Z, Youn HS, Lee WH, Zhao L, et al. Reciprocal modulation of toll-like receptor-4 signaling pathways involving MyD88 and phosphatidylinositol 3-kinase/AKT by saturated and polyunsaturated fatty acids. The Journal of Biological Chemistry. 2003;**278**(39):37041-37051

[63] Chen A, Mumick S, Zhang C, Lamb J, Dai H, Weingarth D, et al. Diet induction of monocyte chemoattractant protein-1 and its impact on obesity. Obesity Research. 2005;**13**(8):1311-1320

[64] Rogers NH, Perfield JW 2nd, Strissel KJ, Obin MS, Greenberg AS. Reduced energy expenditure and increased inflammation are early events in the development of ovariectomy-induced obesity. Endocrinology. 2009;**150**(5):2161-2168

[65] Sartipy P, Loskutoff DJ. Monocyte chemoattractant protein 1 in obesity and insulin resistance. Proceedings of the National Academy of Sciences of the United States of America. 2003;**100**(12):7265-7270

[66] Muscogiuri G, Pugliese G, Laudisio D, Castellucci B, Barrea L, Savastano S, et al. The impact of obesity on immune response to infection: Plausible mechanisms and outcomes. Obesity Reviews. 2021;**22**(6):e13216

[67] Falagas ME, Kompoti M. Obesity and infection. The Lancet Infectious Diseases. 2006;**6**(7):438-446

[68] O'Shea D, Corrigan M, Dunne MR, Jackson R, Woods C, Gaoatswe G, et al. Changes in human dendritic cell number and function in severe obesity may contribute to increased susceptibility to viral infection. International Journal of Obesity. 2013;**37**(11):1510-1513

[69] Wacharasint P, Boyd JH, Russell JA, Walley KR. One size does not fit all in severe infection: Obesity alters outcome, susceptibility, treatment, and inflammatory response. Critical Care. 2013;**17**(3):R122

[70] O'Sullivan KE, Reynolds JV, O'Hanlon C, O'Sullivan JN, Lysaght J. Could signal transducer and activator of transcription 3 be a therapeutic target in obesity-related gastrointestinal malignancy? Journal of Gastrointestinal Cancer. 2014;**45**(1):1-11

[71] Chien Y, Scuoppo C, Wang X, Fang X, Balgley B, Bolden JE, et al. Control of the senescence-associated secretory phenotype by NF-kappaB promotes senescence and enhances chemosensitivity. Genes and Development. 2011;**25**(20): 2125-2136

[72] Huber MA, Azoitei N, Baumann B, Grunert S, Sommer A, Pehamberger H, et al. NF-kappaB is essential for epithelial-mesenchymal transition and metastasis in a model of breast cancer progression. The Journal of Clinical Investigation. 2004;**114**(4):569-581

[73] Elinav E, Nowarski R, Thaiss CA, Hu B, Jin C, Flavell RA. Inflammation-induced cancer: Crosstalk between

tumours, immune cells and microorganisms. Nature Reviews. Cancer. 2013;**13**(11):759-771

[74] Gonzalez-Cantero J, Martin-Rodriguez JL, Gonzalez-Cantero A, Arrebola JP, Gonzalez-Calvin JL. Insulin resistance in lean and overweight non-diabetic Caucasian adults: Study of its relationship with liver triglyceride content, waist circumference and BMI. PLoS One. 2018;**13**(2):e0192663

[75] Esposito K, Chiodini P, Colao A, Lenzi A, Giugliano D. Metabolic syndrome and risk of cancer: A systematic review and meta-analysis. Diabetes Care. 2012;**35**(11):2402-2411

[76] Dimitriadis G, Mitrou P, Lambadiari V, Maratou E, Raptis SA. Insulin effects in muscle and adipose tissue. Diabetes Research and Clinical Practice. 2011;**93**(Suppl. 1): S52-S59

[77] Saponaro C, Gaggini M, Carli F, Gastaldelli A. The subtle balance between lipolysis and lipogenesis: A critical point in metabolic homeostasis. Nutrients. 2015;**7**(11):9453-9474

[78] Girousse A, Tavernier G, Valle C, Moro C, Mejhert N, Dinel AL, et al. Partial inhibition of adipose tissue lipolysis improves glucose metabolism and insulin sensitivity without alteration of fat mass. PLoS Biology. 2013;**11**(2):e1001485

[79] Hale JS, Otvos B, Sinyuk M, Alvarado AG, Hitomi M, Stoltz K, et al. Cancer stem cell-specific scavenger receptor CD36 drives glioblastoma progression. Stem Cells. 2014;**32**(7):1746-1758

[80] Ladanyi A, Mukherjee A, Kenny HA, Johnson A, Mitra AK, Sundaresan S, et al. Adipocyte-induced CD36 expression drives ovarian cancer progression and metastasis. Oncogene. 2018;**37**(17):2285-2301

[81] Feng WW, Wilkins O, Bang S, Ung M, Li J, An J, et al. CD36-mediated metabolic rewiring of breast cancer cells promotes resistance to HER2-targeted therapies. Cell Reports. 2019;**29**(11):3405-20 e5

[82] Pan J, Fan Z, Wang Z, Dai Q, Xiang Z, Yuan F, et al. CD36 mediates palmitate acid-induced metastasis of gastric cancer via AKT/GSK-3β/β-catenin pathway. Journal of Experimental and Clinical Cancer Research. 2019;**38**(1):52

[83] Cai L, Wang Z, Ji A, Meyer JM, van der Westhuyzen DR. Scavenger receptor CD36 expression contributes to adipose tissue inflammation and cell death in diet-induced obesity. PLoS One. 2012;**7**(5):e36785

[84] Yang P, Qin H, Li Y, Xiao A, Zheng E, Zeng H, et al. CD36-mediated metabolic crosstalk between tumor cells and macrophages affects liver metastasis. Nature Communications. 2022;**13**(1):5782

[85] Zhu GQ, Tang Z, Huang R, Qu WF, Fang Y, Yang R, et al. CD36(+) cancer-associated fibroblasts provide immunosuppressive microenvironment for hepatocellular carcinoma via secretion of macrophage migration inhibitory factor. Cell Discovery. 2023;**9**(1):25

[86] MacDougald OA, Burant CF. The rapidly expanding family of adipokines. Cell Metabolism. 2007;**6**(3):159-161

[87] Scherer PE, Williams S, Fogliano M, Baldini G, Lodish HF. A novel serum protein similar to C1q, produced exclusively in adipocytes.

The Journal of Biological Chemistry. 1995;**270**(45):26746-26749

[88] Schilling JD, Machkovech HM, He L, Sidhu R, Fujiwara H, Weber K, et al. Palmitate and lipopolysaccharide trigger synergistic ceramide production in primary macrophages. The Journal of Biological Chemistry. 2013;**288**(5):2923-2932

[89] Okazaki R, Inoue D, Shibata M, Saika M, Kido S, Ooka H, et al. Estrogen promotes early osteoblast differentiation and inhibits adipocyte differentiation in mouse bone marrow stromal cell lines that express estrogen receptor (ER) α or β. Endocrinology. 2002;**143**(6):2349-2356

[90] Hong L, Colpan A, Peptan IA, Daw J, George A, Evans CA. 17-β Estradiol enhances osteogenic and adipogenic differentiation of human adipose-derived stromal cells. Tissue Engineering. 2007;**13**(6):1197-1203

[91] Bouchard C, Després JP, Mauriège P. Genetic and nongenetic determinants of regional fat distribution. Endocrine Reviews. 1993;**14**(1):72-93

[92] Garaulet M, Pérez-Llamas F, Baraza JC, Garcia-Prieto MD, Fardy PS, Tébar FJ, et al. Body fat distribution in pre-and post-menopausal women: Metabolic and anthropometric variables. The Journal of Nutrition, Health and Aging. 2002;**6**(2):123-126

[93] Clusan L, Ferrière F, Flouriot G, Pakdel F. A basic review on estrogen receptor signaling pathways in breast cancer. International Journal of Molecular Sciences. 2023;**24**(7)

[94] Barton M, Filardo EJ, Lolait SJ, Thomas P, Maggiolini M, Prossnitz ER. Twenty years of the G protein-coupled estrogen receptor GPER: Historical and personal perspectives. The Journal of Steroid Biochemistry and Molecular Biology. 2018;**176**:4-15

[95] Kelly MJ, Levin ER. Rapid actions of plasma membrane estrogen receptors. Trends in Endocrinology and Metabolism. 2001;**12**(4):152-156

[96] Donegan WL, Johnstone MF, Biedrzycki L. Obesity, estrogen production, and tumor estrogen receptors in women with carcinoma of the breast. American Journal of Clinical Oncology. 1983;**6**(1):19-24

[97] Baglietto L, English DR, Hopper JL, MacInnis RJ, Morris HA, Tilley WD, et al. Circulating steroid hormone concentrations in postmenopausal women in relation to body size and composition. Breast Cancer Research and Treatment. 2009;**115**(1):171-179

[98] Zhao Y, Nichols JE, Valdez R, Mendelson CR, Simpson ER. Tumor necrosis factor-alpha stimulates aromatase gene expression in human adipose stromal cells through use of an activating protein-1 binding site upstream of promoter 1.4. Molecular Endocrinology. 1996;**10**(11):1350-1357

[99] Bowers LW, Brenner AJ, Hursting SD, Tekmal RR, deGraffenried LA. Obesity-associated systemic interleukin-6 promotes pre-adipocyte aromatase expression via increased breast cancer cell prostaglandin E2 production. Breast Cancer Research and Treatment. 2015;**149**(1):49-57

[100] Brown KA, McInnes KJ, Hunger NI, Oakhill JS, Steinberg GR, Simpson ER. Subcellular localization of cyclic AMP-responsive element binding protein-regulated transcription coactivator 2 provides a link between obesity and breast cancer in postmenopausal women. Cancer Research. 2009;**69**(13):5392-5399

[101] Bulun SE, Sharda G, Rink J, Sharma S, Simpson ER. Distribution of aromatase P450 transcripts and adipose fibroblasts in the human breast. The Journal of Clinical Endocrinology and Metabolism. 1996;**81**(3):1273-1277

[102] Gusberg SB. Precursors of corpus carcinoma estrogens and adenomatous hyperplasia. American Journal of Obstetrics and Gynecology. 1947;**54**(6):905-927

[103] Bokhman JV. Two pathogenetic types of endometrial carcinoma. Gynecologic Oncology. 1983;**15**(1):10-17

[104] Rodriguez AC, Blanchard Z, Maurer KA, Gertz J. Estrogen signaling in endometrial cancer: A key oncogenic pathway with several open questions. Hormones and Cancer. 2019;**10**(2-3):51-63

[105] Bartosch C, Monteiro-Reis S, Vieira R, Pereira A, Rodrigues M, Jerónimo C, et al. Endometrial endometrioid carcinoma metastases show decreased ER-alpha and PR-A expression compared to matched primary tumors. PLoS One. 2015;**10**(8):e0134969

[106] Webb PM. Obesity and gynecologic cancer etiology and survival. American Society of Clinical Oncology Educational Book. 2013;**33**:e222-e2e8

[107] Rivera-Izquierdo M, Pérez de Rojas J, Martínez-Ruiz V, Pérez-Gómez B, Sánchez MJ, Khan KS, et al. Obesity as a risk factor for prostate cancer mortality: A systematic review and dose-response meta-analysis of 280,199 patients. Cancers (Basel). 2021;**13**(16)

[108] Petrelli F, Cortellini A, Indini A, Tomasello G, Ghidini M, Nigro O, et al. Association of obesity with survival outcomes in patients with cancer: A systematic review and meta-analysis. JAMA Network Open. 2021;**4**(3):e213520-e21352e

[109] Smith SR. The endocrinology of obesity. Endocrinology and Metabolism Clinics of North America. 1996;**25**(4):921-942

[110] Kirschner MA, Samojlik E, Drejka M, Szmal E, Schneider G, Ertel N. Androgen-estrogen metabolism in women with upper body versus lower body obesity. The Journal of Clinical Endocrinology and Metabolism. 1990;**70**(2):473-479

[111] Joly-Pharaboz MO, Soave MC, Nicolas B, Mebarki F, Renaud M, Foury O, et al. Androgens inhibit the proliferation of a variant of the human prostate cancer cell line LNCaP. The Journal of Steroid Biochemistry and Molecular Biology. 1995;**55**(1):67-76

[112] Heisler LE, Evangelou A, Lew AM, Trachtenberg J, Elsholtz HP, Brown TJ. Androgen-dependent cell cycle arrest and apoptotic death in PC-3 prostatic cell cultures expressing a full-length human androgen receptor. Molecular and Cellular Endocrinology. 1997;**126**(1):59-73

[113] Lamont KR, Tindall DJ. Minireview: Alternative activation pathways for the androgen receptor in prostate cancer. Molecular Endocrinology. 2011;**25**(6):897-907

[114] Nakashima J, Tachibana M, Horiguchi Y, Oya M, Ohigashi T, Asakura H, et al. Serum interleukin 6 as a prognostic factor in patients with prostate cancer. Clinical Cancer Research. 2000;**6**(7):2702-2706

[115] Degeorges A, Tatoud R, Fauvel-Lafeve F, Podgorniak MP, Millot G, de Cremoux P, et al. Stromal cells from

human benign prostate hyperplasia produce a growth-inhibitory factor for LNCaP prostate cancer cells, identified as interleukin-6. International Journal of Cancer. 1996;**68**(2):207-214

[116] Chen T, Wang LH, Farrar WL. Interleukin 6 activates androgen receptor-mediated gene expression through a signal transducer and activator of transcription 3-dependent pathway in LNCaP prostate cancer cells. Cancer Research. 2000;**60**(8):2132-2135

[117] Malinowska K, Neuwirt H, Cavarretta IT, Bektic J, Steiner H, Dietrich H, et al. Interleukin-6 stimulation of growth of prostate cancer in vitro and in vivo through activation of the androgen receptor. Endocrine-Related Cancer. 2009;**16**(1):155-169

[118] Hobisch A, Eder IE, Putz T, Horninger W, Bartsch G, Klocker H, et al. Interleukin-6 regulates prostate-specific protein expression in prostate carcinoma cells by activation of the androgen receptor. Cancer Research. 1998;**58**(20):4640-4645

[119] Handle F, Puhr M, Schaefer G, Lorito N, Hoefer J, Gruber M, et al. The STAT3 inhibitor galiellalactone reduces IL6-mediated AR activity in benign and malignant prostate models. Molecular Cancer Therapeutics. 2018;**17**(12):2722-2731

[120] Seaton A, Scullin P, Maxwell PJ, Wilson C, Pettigrew J, Gallagher R, et al. Interleukin-8 signaling promotes androgen-independent proliferation of prostate cancer cells via induction of androgen receptor expression and activation. Carcinogenesis. 2008;**29**(6):1148-1156

[121] Zurita-Cruz JN, Villasís-Keever MA, Manuel-Apolinar L, Damasio-Santana L, Garrido-Magaña E, Rivera-Hernández AJ. Leptin/adiponectin ratio as a prognostic factor for increased weight gain in girls with central precocious puberty. Frontiers in Endocrinology (Lausanne). 2023;**14**:1101399

[122] Senkus KE, Crowe-White KM, Bolland AC, Locher JL, Ard JD. Changes in adiponectin: Leptin ratio among older adults with obesity following a 12-month exercise and diet intervention. Nutrition and Diabetes. 2022;**12**(1):30

[123] Margetic S, Gazzola C, Pegg GG, Hill RA. Leptin: A review of its peripheral actions and interactions. International Journal of Obesity and Related Metabolic Disorders. 2002;**26**(11):1407-1433

[124] Bjorbaek C, Kahn BB. Leptin signaling in the central nervous system and the periphery. Recent Progress in Hormone Research. 2004;**59**:305-331

[125] Yu F, Fu R, Liu L, Wang X, Wu T, Shen W, et al. Leptin-induced angiogenesis of EA.Hy926 endothelial cells via the Akt and Wnt signaling pathways in vitro and in vivo. Frontiers in Pharmacology. 2019;**10**:1275

[126] Obradovic M, Sudar-Milovanovic E, Soskic S, Essack M, Arya S, Stewart AJ, et al. Leptin and obesity: Role and clinical implication. Frontiers in Endocrinology (Lausanne). 2021;**12**:585887

[127] Klein S, Coppack SW, Mohamed-Ali V, Landt M. Adipose tissue leptin production and plasma leptin kinetics in humans. Diabetes. 1996;**45**(7): 984-987

[128] Zhou Y, Rui L. Leptin signaling and leptin resistance. Frontiers in Medicine. 2013;**7**(2):207-222

[129] Onuma M, Bub JD, Rummel TL, Iwamoto Y. Prostate cancer

cell-adipocyte interaction: Leptin mediates androgen-independent prostate cancer cell proliferation through c-Jun NH2-terminal kinase. The Journal of Biological Chemistry. 2003;**278**(43):42660-42667

[130] Ptak A, Kolaczkowska E, Gregoraszczuk EL. Leptin stimulation of cell cycle and inhibition of apoptosis gene and protein expression in OVCAR-3 ovarian cancer cells. Endocrine. 2013;**43**(2):394-403

[131] Liu Y, Lv L, Xiao W, Gong C, Yin J, Wang D, et al. Leptin activates STAT3 and ERK1/2 pathways and induces endometrial cancer cell proliferation. Journal of Huazhong University of Science and Technology. Medical Sciences. 2011;**31**(3):365

[132] Strong AL, Strong TA, Rhodes LV, Semon JA, Zhang X, Shi Z, et al. Obesity associated alterations in the biology of adipose stem cells mediate enhanced tumorigenesis by estrogen dependent pathways. Breast Cancer Research. 2013;**15**(5):R102

[133] Mishra AK, Parish CR, Wong ML, Licinio J, Blackburn AC. Leptin signals via TGFB1 to promote metastatic potential and stemness in breast cancer. PLoS One. 2017;**12**(5):e0178454

[134] Xu CJ, Dong LL, Kang XL, Li ZM, Zhang HY. Leptin promotes proliferation and inhibits apoptosis of prostate cancer cells by regulating ERK1/2 signaling pathway. European Review for Medical and Pharmacological Sciences. 2020;**24**(16):8341-8348

[135] Haque I, Ghosh A, Acup S, Banerjee S, Dhar K, Ray A, et al. Leptin-induced ER-α-positive breast cancer cell viability and migration is mediated by suppressing CCN5-signaling via activating JAK/AKT/STAT-pathway. BMC Cancer. 2018;**18**(1):99

[136] Fan Y, Gan Y, Shen Y, Cai X, Song Y, Zhao F, et al. Leptin signaling enhances cell invasion and promotes the metastasis of human pancreatic cancer via increasing MMP-13 production. Oncotarget. 2015;**6**(18):16120-16134

[137] Cao R, Brakenhielm E, Wahlestedt C, Thyberg J, Cao Y. Leptin induces vascular permeability and synergistically stimulates angiogenesis with FGF-2 and VEGF. Proceedings of the National Academy of Sciences of the United States of America. 2001;**98**(11):6390-6395

[138] Esper RM, Dame M, McClintock S, Holt PR, Dannenberg AJ, Wicha MS, et al. Leptin and adiponectin modulate the self-renewal of normal human breast epithelial stem cells. Cancer Prevention Research (Philadelphia, Pa.). 2015;**8**(12):1174-1183

[139] Harbuzariu A, Rampoldi A, Daley-Brown DS, Candelaria P, Harmon TL, Lipsey CC, et al. Leptin-notch signaling axis is involved in pancreatic cancer progression. Oncotarget. 2017;**8**(5):7740-7752

[140] Obi N, Jung AY, Maurer T, Huebner M, Johnson T, Behrens S, et al. Association of circulating leptin, adiponectin, and resistin concentrations with long-term breast cancer prognosis in a German patient cohort. Scientific Reports. 2021;**11**(1):23526

[141] Kwiatkowska K, Rhone P, Wrzeszcz K, Ruszkowska-Ciastek B. High post-treatment leptin concentration as a prognostic biomarker of the high risk of luminal breast cancer relapse: A six-year comprehensive study. Life (Basel). 2022;**12**(12)

[142] Li C, Quan J, Wei R, Zhao Z, Guan X, Liu Z, et al. Leptin overexpression as a poor prognostic

factor for colorectal cancer. BioMed Research International. 2020;**2020**:7532514

[143] Bavi P, Ahmed M, Devarajan S, Moorji A, Atizado V, Balde V, et al. Leptin-R is an independent prognostic marker in colorectal carcinoma. Cancer Research. 2008;**988**

[144] Wu MH, Chou YC, Chou WY, Hsu GC, Chu CH, Yu CP, et al. Circulating levels of leptin, adiposity and breast cancer risk. British Journal of Cancer. 2009;**100**(4):578-582

[145] Arita Y, Kihara S, Ouchi N, Takahashi M, Maeda K, Miyagawa J, et al. Paradoxical decrease of an adipose-specific protein, adiponectin, in obesity. Biochemical and Biophysical Research Communications. 1999;**257**(1):79-83

[146] Kopp HP, Krzyzanowska K, Mohlig M, Spranger J, Pfeiffer AF, Schernthaner G. Effects of marked weight loss on plasma levels of adiponectin, markers of chronic subclinical inflammation and insulin resistance in morbidly obese women. International Journal of Obesity. 2005;**29**(7):766-771

[147] Yu Z, Tang S, Ma H, Duan H, Zeng Y. Association of serum adiponectin with breast cancer: A meta-analysis of 27 case-control studies. Medicine. 2019;**98**(6):e14359

[148] Korner A, Pazaitou-Panayiotou K, Kelesidis T, Kelesidis I, Williams CJ, Kaprara A, et al. Total and high-molecular-weight adiponectin in breast cancer: in vitro and in vivo studies. The Journal of Clinical Endocrinology and Metabolism. 2007;**92**(3):1041-1048

[149] Otokozawa S, Tanaka R, Akasaka H, Ito E, Asakura S, Ohnishi H, et al. Associations of serum isoflavone, adiponectin and insulin levels with risk for epithelial ovarian cancer: Results of a case-control study. Asian Pacific Journal of Cancer Prevention. 2015;**16**(12):4987-4991

[150] Li H, Sun L, Chen L, Kang Z, Hao G, Bai F. Effects of adiponectin, plasma D-dimer, inflammation and tumor markers on clinical characteristics and prognosis of patients with ovarian cancer. Journal Of Medical Biochemistry. 2022;**41**(1):71-78

[151] Burton AJ, Gilbert R, Tilling K, Langdon R, Donovan JL, Holly JMP, et al. Circulating adiponectin and leptin and risk of overall and aggressive prostate cancer: A systematic review and meta-analysis. Scientific Reports. 2021;**11**(1):320

[152] Michalakis K, Williams CJ, Mitsiades N, Blakeman J, Balafouta-Tselenis S, Giannopoulos A, et al. Serum adiponectin concentrations and tissue expression of adiponectin receptors are reduced in patients with prostate cancer: A case control study. Cancer Epidemiology, Biomarkers and Prevention. 2007;**16**(2):308-313

[153] Wei T, Ye P, Peng X, Wu LL, Yu GY. Circulating adiponectin levels in various malignancies: An updated meta-analysis of 107 studies. Oncotarget. 2016;**7**(30):48671-48691

[154] Miyoshi Y, Funahashi T, Kihara S, Taguchi T, Tamaki Y, Matsuzawa Y, et al. Association of serum adiponectin levels with breast cancer risk. Clinical Cancer Research. 2003;**9**(15):5699-5704

[155] Kim AY, Lee YS, Kim KH, Lee JH, Lee HK, Jang S-H, et al. Adiponectin represses colon cancer cell proliferation via AdipoR1- and -R2-mediated AMPK activation. Molecular Endocrinology. 2010;**24**(7):1441-1452

[156] Man K, Ng KT, Xu A, Cheng Q, Lo CM, Xiao JW, et al. Suppression of liver tumor growth and metastasis by adiponectin in nude mice through inhibition of tumor angiogenesis and downregulation of rho kinase/IFN-inducible protein 10/matrix metalloproteinase 9 signaling. Clinical Cancer Research. 2010;**16**(3):967-977

[157] Wang Y, Lam JB, Lam KS, Liu J, Lam MC, Hoo RL, et al. Adiponectin modulates the glycogen synthase kinase-3beta/beta-catenin signaling pathway and attenuates mammary tumorigenesis of MDA-MB-231 cells in nude mice. Cancer Research. 2006;**66**(23):11462-11470

[158] Ishikawa M, Kitayama J, Yamauchi T, Kadowaki T, Maki T, Miyato H, et al. Adiponectin inhibits the growth and peritoneal metastasis of gastric cancer through its specific membrane receptors AdipoR1 and AdipoR2. Cancer Science. 2007;**98**(7):1120-1127

[159] Chiu YC, Shieh DC, Tong KM, Chen CP, Huang KC, Chen PC, et al. Involvement of AdipoR receptor in adiponectin-induced motility and alpha2beta1 integrin upregulation in human chondrosarcoma cells. Carcinogenesis. 2009;**30**(10):1651-1659

[160] Takahata C, Miyoshi Y, Irahara N, Taguchi T, Tamaki Y, Noguchi S. Demonstration of adiponectin receptors 1 and 2 mRNA expression in human breast cancer cells. Cancer Letters. 2007;**250**(2):229-236

[161] Chou SH, Tseleni-Balafouta S, Moon HS, Chamberland JP, Liu X, Kavantzas N, et al. Adiponectin receptor expression in human malignant tissues. Hormones and Cancer. 2010;**1**(3):136-145

[162] Luo Z, Saha AK, Xiang X, Ruderman NB. AMPK, the metabolic syndrome and cancer. Trends in Pharmacological Sciences. 2005;**26**(2):69-76

[163] Nakayama S, Miyoshi Y, Ishihara H, Noguchi S. Growth-inhibitory effect of adiponectin via adiponectin receptor 1 on human breast cancer cells through inhibition of S-phase entry without inducing apoptosis. Breast Cancer Research and Treatment. 2008;**112**(3):405-410

[164] Dos Santos E, Benaitreau D, Dieudonne M-N, Leneveu M-C, Serazin V, Giudicelli Y, et al. Adiponectin mediates an antiproliferative response in human MDA-MB 231 breast cancer cells. Oncology Reports. 2008;**20**(4):971-977

[165] Konturek PC, Burnat G, Rau T, Hahn EG, Konturek S. Effect of adiponectin and ghrelin on apoptosis of Barrett adenocarcinoma cell line. Digestive Diseases and Sciences. 2008;**53**(3):597-605

[166] Saxena NK, Fu PP, Nagalingam A, Wang J, Handy J, Cohen C, et al. Adiponectin modulates C-Jun N-terminal kinase and mammalian target of rapamycin and inhibits hepatocellular carcinoma. Gastroenterology. 2010;**139**(5):1762-1773, 73 e1-5

[167] Bråkenhielm E, Veitonmäki N, Cao R, Kihara S, Matsuzawa Y, Zhivotovsky B, et al. Adiponectin-induced antiangiogenesis and antitumor activity involve caspase-mediated endothelial cell apoptosis. Proceedings of the National Academy of Sciences of the United States of America. 2004;**101**(8):2476-2481

[168] Cong L, Gasser J, Zhao J, Yang B, Li F, Zhao AZ. Human adiponectin inhibits cell growth and induces apoptosis in human endometrial carcinoma cells, HEC-1-a and RL95 2. Endocrine-Related Cancer. 2007;**14**(3):713-720

[169] Wang Y, Lam KS, Xu JY, Lu G, Xu LY, Cooper GJ, et al. Adiponectin inhibits cell proliferation by interacting with several growth factors in an oligomerization-dependent manner. The Journal of Biological Chemistry. 2005;**280**(18):18341-18347

[170] Arita Y, Kihara S, Ouchi N, Maeda K, Kuriyama H, Okamoto Y, et al. Adipocyte-derived plasma protein adiponectin acts as a platelet-derived growth factor-BB-binding protein and regulates growth factor-induced common postreceptor signal in vascular smooth muscle cell. Circulation. 2002;**105**(24):2893-2898

[171] Čolak E, Pap D. The role of oxidative stress in the development of obesity and obesity-related metabolic disorders. Journal Of Medical Biochemistry. 2021;**40**(1):1-9

[172] Furukawa S, Fujita T, Shimabukuro M, Iwaki M, Yamada Y, Nakajima Y, et al. Increased oxidative stress in obesity and its impact on metabolic syndrome. The Journal of Clinical Investigation. 2004;**114**(12):1752-1761

[173] Leanza G, Conte C, Cannata F, Isgrò C, Piccoli A, Strollo R, et al. Oxidative stress in postmenopausal women with or without obesity. Cells. 2023;**12**(8)

[174] Den Hartigh LJ, Omer M, Goodspeed L, Wang S, Wietecha T, O'Brien KD, et al. Adipocyte-specific deficiency of NADPH oxidase 4 delays the onset of insulin resistance and attenuates adipose tissue inflammation in obesity. Arteriosclerosis, Thrombosis, and Vascular Biology. 2017;**37**(3):466-475

[175] Morita Y, Senokuchi T, Yamada S, Wada T, Furusho T, Matsumura T, et al. Impact of tissue macrophage proliferation on peripheral and systemic insulin resistance in obese mice with diabetes. BMJ Open Diabetes Research and Care. 2020;**8**(1):e001578

[176] Oliveira-Marques V, Marinho HS, Cyrne L, Antunes F. Role of hydrogen peroxide in NF-kappaB activation: From inducer to modulator. Antioxidants and Redox Signaling. 2009;**11**(9):2223-2243

[177] Nomura M, Ma W, Chen N, Bode AM, Dong Z. Inhibition of 12-O-tetradecanoylphorbol-13-acetate-induced NF-kappaB activation by tea polyphenols, (−)-epigallocatechin gallate and theaflavins. Carcinogenesis. 2000;**21**(10):1885-1890

[178] Chandel NS, Trzyna WC, McClintock DS, Schumacker PT. Role of oxidants in NF-kappa B activation and TNF-alpha gene transcription induced by hypoxia and endotoxin. Journal of Immunology. 2000;**165**(2):1013-1021

[179] Schreck R, Meier B, Männel DN, Dröge W, Baeuerle PA. Dithiocarbamates as potent inhibitors of nuclear factor kappa B activation in intact cells. The Journal of Experimental Medicine. 1992;**175**(5):1181-1194

[180] Shin DH, Dier U, Melendez JA, Hempel N. Regulation of MMP-1 expression in response to hypoxia is dependent on the intracellular redox status of metastatic bladder cancer cells. Biochimica et Biophysica Acta. 2015;**1852**(12):2593-2602

[181] Liu Y, Cui Y, Shi M, Zhang Q, Wang Q, Chen X. Deferoxamine promotes MDA-MB-231 cell migration and invasion through increased ROS-dependent HIF-1α accumulation. Cellular Physiology and Biochemistry. 2014;**33**(4):1036-1046

[182] Xia C, Meng Q, Liu LZ, Rojanasakul Y, Wang XR, Jiang BH.

Reactive oxygen species regulate angiogenesis and tumor growth through vascular endothelial growth factor. Cancer Research. 2007;**67**(22):10823-10830

[183] Dirat B, Bochet L, Dabek M, Daviaud D, Dauvillier S, Majed B, et al. Cancer-associated adipocytes exhibit an activated phenotype and contribute to breast cancer invasion. Cancer Research. 2011;**71**(7):2455-2465

[184] Bochet L, Lehuédé C, Dauvillier S, Wang YY, Dirat B, Laurent V, et al. Adipocyte-derived fibroblasts promote tumor progression and contribute to the desmoplastic reaction in breast cancer. Cancer Research. 2013;**73**(18):5657-5668

[185] Zoico E, Darra E, Rizzatti V, Budui S, Franceschetti G, Mazzali G, et al. Adipocytes WNT5a mediated dedifferentiation: A possible target in pancreatic cancer microenvironment. Oncotarget. 2016;7(15):20223-20235

[186] Song Y, Na H, Lee SE, Kim YM, Moon J, Nam TW, et al. Dysfunctional adipocytes promote tumor progression through YAP/TAZ-dependent cancer-associated adipocyte transformation. Nature Communications. 2024;**15**(1):4052

[187] Wang YY, Attané C, Milhas D, Dirat B, Dauvillier S, Guerard A, et al. Mammary adipocytes stimulate breast cancer invasion through metabolic remodeling of tumor cells. JCI Insight. 2017;**2**(4):e87489

[188] von Gruenigen VE, Tian C, Frasure H, Waggoner S, Keys H, Barakat RR. Treatment effects, disease recurrence, and survival in obese women with early endometrial carcinoma : A gynecologic oncology group study. Cancer. 2006;**107**(12):2786-2791

[189] Kroenke CH, Chen WY, Rosner B, Holmes MD. Weight, weight gain, and survival after breast cancer diagnosis. Journal of Clinical Oncology. 2005;**23**(7):1370-1378

[190] Meyerhardt JA, Catalano PJ, Haller DG, Mayer RJ, Benson AB 3rd, Macdonald JS, et al. Influence of body mass index on outcomes and treatment-related toxicity in patients with colon carcinoma. Cancer. 2003;**98**(3):484-495

[191] Gross JP, Strauss JB, Lurain J, Berry E, Neubauer N, Helenowski I, et al. Impact of obesity on treatment-related adverse events, disease recurrence, and survival in women with cervical carcinoma. Journal of Radiation Oncology. 2016;**5**(2):197-203

[192] Helyer LK, Varnic M, Le LW, Leong W, McCready D. Obesity is a risk factor for developing postoperative lymphedema in breast cancer patients. The Breast Journal. 2010;**16**(1):48-54

[193] World Cancer Research Fund/ American Institute for Cancer Research. Diet, Nutrition, Physical Activity and Cancer: A Global Perspective. Continuous Update Project Expert Report. 2018. Available from: https://www.wcrf.org/wp-content/uploads/2024/11/Summary-of-Third-Expert-Report-2018.pdf

[194] Malcomson FC, Wiggins C, Parra-Soto S, Ho FK, Celis-Morales C, Sharp L, et al. Adherence to the 2018 World Cancer Research Fund/American Institute for Cancer Research Cancer prevention recommendations and cancer risk: A systematic review and meta-analysis. Cancer. 2023;**129**(17):2655-2670

[195] Coppola A, Marfella R, Coppola L, Tagliamonte E, Fontana D, Liguori E, et al. Effect of weight loss on coronary circulation and adiponectin levels in

obese women. International Journal of Cardiology. 2009;**134**(3):414-416

[196] Coughlin CC, Finck BN, Eagon JC, Halpin VJ, Magkos F, Mohammed BS, et al. Effect of marked weight loss on adiponectin gene expression and plasma concentrations. Obesity (Silver Spring). 2007;**15**(3):640-645

[197] Crujeiras AB, Goyenechea E, Abete I, Lage M, Carreira MC, Martinez JA, et al. Weight regain after a diet-induced loss is predicted by higher baseline leptin and lower ghrelin plasma levels. The Journal of Clinical Endocrinology and Metabolism. 2010;**95**(11):5037-5044

[198] Pardina E, Ferrer R, Baena-Fustegueras JA, Lecube A, Fort JM, Vargas V, et al. The relationships between IGF-1 and CRP, NO, leptin, and adiponectin during weight loss in the morbidly obese. Obesity Surgery. 2010;**20**(5):623-632

[199] Reinehr T, Roth C, Menke T, Andler W. Adiponectin before and after weight loss in obese children. The Journal of Clinical Endocrinology and Metabolism. 2004;**89**(8):3790-3794

[200] Rolland C, Hession M, Broom I. Effect of weight loss on adipokine levels in obese patients. Diabetes, Metabolic Syndrome and Obesity. 2011;**4**:315-323

[201] Soni AC, Conroy MB, Mackey RH, Kuller LH. Ghrelin, leptin, adiponectin, and insulin levels and concurrent and future weight change in overweight, postmenopausal women. Menopause. 2011;**18**(3):296-301

[202] Campbell KL, Foster-Schubert KE, Alfano CM, Wang CC, Wang CY, Duggan CR, et al. Reduced-calorie dietary weight loss, exercise, and sex hormones in postmenopausal women: Randomized controlled trial. Journal of Clinical Oncology. 2012;**30**(19):2314-2326

[203] Kaaks R, Bellati C, Venturelli E, Rinaldi S, Secreto G, Biessy C, et al. Effects of dietary intervention on IGF-I and IGF-binding proteins, and related alterations in sex steroid metabolism: The diet and androgens (DIANA) randomised trial. European Journal of Clinical Nutrition. 2003;**57**(9):1079-1088

[204] Petelin A, Bizjak M, Cernelic-Bizjak M, Jurdana M, Jakus T, Jenko-Praznikar Z. Low-grade inflammation in overweight and obese adults is affected by weight loss program. Journal of Endocrinological Investigation. 2014;**37**(8):745-755

[205] Tchernof A, Nolan A, Sites CK, Ades PA, Poehlman ET. Weight loss reduces C-reactive protein levels in obese postmenopausal women. Circulation. 2002;**105**(5):564-569

[206] Zamarron BF, Mergian TA, Cho KW, Martinez-Santibanez G, Luan D, Singer K, et al. Macrophage proliferation sustains adipose tissue inflammation in formerly obese mice. Diabetes. 2017;**66**(2):392-406

[207] Aleman JO, Iyengar NM, Walker JM, Milne GL, Da Rosa JC, Liang Y, et al. Effects of rapid weight loss on systemic and adipose tissue inflammation and metabolism in obese postmenopausal women. Journal of the Endocrine Society. 2017;**1**(6):625-637

[208] Sramkova V, Rossmeislova L, Krauzova E, Kracmerova J, Koc M, Langin D, et al. Comparison of early (2 days) and later (28 days) response of adipose tissue to very low-calorie diet in obese women. The Journal of Clinical Endocrinology and Metabolism. 2016;**101**(12):5021-5029

[209] Petersen AM, Pedersen BK. The anti-inflammatory effect of exercise. Journal of Applied Physiology (1985). 2005;**98**(4):1154-1162

[210] Steensberg A, Fischer CP, Keller C, Moller K, Pedersen BK. IL-6 enhances plasma IL-1ra, IL-10, and cortisol in humans. American Journal of Physiology. Endocrinology and Metabolism. 2003;**285**(2):E433-E437

[211] Fiers W. Tumor necrosis factor. Characterization at the molecular, cellular and in vivo level. FEBS Letters. 1991;**285**(2):199-212

[212] Kelly M, Keller C, Avilucea PR, Keller P, Luo Z, Xiang X, et al. AMPK activity is diminished in tissues of IL-6 knockout mice: The effect of exercise. Biochemical and Biophysical Research Communications. 2004;**320**(2):449-454

[213] Matthys P, Mitera T, Heremans H, Van Damme J, Billiau A. Anti-gamma interferon and anti-interleukin-6 antibodies affect staphylococcal enterotoxin B-induced weight loss, hypoglycemia, and cytokine release in D-galactosamine-sensitized and unsensitized mice. Infection and Immunity. 1995;**63**(4):1158-1164

[214] Mizuhara H, O'Neill E, Seki N, Ogawa T, Kusunoki C, Otsuka K, et al. T cell activation-associated hepatic injury: Mediation by tumor necrosis factors and protection by interleukin 6. The Journal of Experimental Medicine. 1994;**179**(5):1529-1537

[215] Baek KW, Kim JH, Yu HS, Kim JS. Adipose tissue macrophage polarization is altered during recovery after exercise: A large-scale flow cytometric study. Current Issues in Molecular Biology. 2024;**46**(2):1308-1317

[216] Peppler WT, Anderson ZG, MacRae LM, MacPherson REK, Wright DC. Habitual physical activity protects against lipopolysaccharide-induced inflammation in mouse adipose tissue. Adipocytes. 2017;**6**(1):1-11

[217] McTiernan A, Friedenreich CM, Katzmarzyk PT, Powell KE, Macko R, Buchner D, et al. Physical activity in cancer prevention and survival: A systematic review. Medicine and Science in Sports and Exercise. 2019;**51**(6):1252-1261

[218] Mason C, Foster-Schubert KE, Imayama I, Kong A, Xiao L, Bain C, et al. Dietary weight loss and exercise effects on insulin resistance in postmenopausal women. American Journal of Preventive Medicine. 2011;**41**(4):366-375

[219] Wang QL, Babic A, Rosenthal MH, Lee AA, Zhang Y, Zhang X, et al. Cancer diagnoses after recent weight loss. Journal of the American Medical Association. 2024;**331**(4):318-328

[220] Birks S, Peeters A, Backholer K, O'Brien P, Brown W. A systematic review of the impact of weight loss on cancer incidence and mortality. Obesity Reviews. 2012;**13**(10):868-891

[221] Wang LS, Murphy CT, Ruth K, Zaorsky NG, Smaldone MC, Sobczak ML, et al. Impact of obesity on outcomes after definitive dose-escalated intensity-modulated radiotherapy for localized prostate cancer. Cancer. 2015;**121**(17):3010-3017

[222] Lennon H, Sperrin M, Badrick E, Renehan AG. The obesity paradox in cancer: A review. Current Oncology Reports. 2016;**18**(9):56

[223] Wang Z, Aguilar EG, Luna JI, Dunai C, Khuat LT, Le CT, et al. Paradoxical effects of obesity on T cell function during tumor progression

and PD-1 checkpoint blockade. Nature Medicine. 2019;**25**(1):141-151

[224] Zhang SS, Yang H, Luo KJ, Huang QY, Chen JY, Yang F, et al. The impact of body mass index on complication and survival in resected oesophageal cancer: A clinical-based cohort and meta-analysis. British Journal of Cancer. 2013;**109**(11):2894-2903

[225] Zhang J, Chen Q, Li ZM, Xu XD, Song AF, Wang LS. Association of body mass index with mortality and postoperative survival in renal cell cancer patients, a meta-analysis. Oncotarget. 2018;**9**(17):13959-13970

[226] Mullen JT, Davenport DL, Hutter MM, Hosokawa PW, Henderson WG, Khuri SF, et al. Impact of body mass index on perioperative outcomes in patients undergoing major intra-abdominal cancer surgery. Annals of Surgical Oncology. 2008;**15**(8):2164-2172

[227] Navarro WH, Loberiza FR Jr, Bajorunaite R, van Besien K, Vose JM, Lazarus HM, et al. Effect of body mass index on mortality of patients with lymphoma undergoing autologous hematopoietic cell transplantation. Biology of Blood and Marrow Transplantation. 2006;**12**(5):541-551

[228] Brunner AM, Sadrzadeh H, Feng Y, Drapkin BJ, Ballen KK, Attar EC, et al. Association between baseline body mass index and overall survival among patients over age 60 with acute myeloid leukemia. American Journal of Hematology. 2013;**88**(8):642-646

[229] Schlesinger S, Siegert S, Koch M, Walter J, Heits N, Hinz S, et al. Postdiagnosis body mass index and risk of mortality in colorectal cancer survivors: A prospective study and meta-analysis. Cancer Causes and Control. 2014;**25**(10):1407-1418

[230] Ferguson MK, Im HK, Watson S, Johnson E, Wigfield CH, Vigneswaran WT. Association of body mass index and outcomes after major lung resection. European Journal of Cardio-Thoracic Surgery. 2014;**45**(4):e94-e99; discussion e9

[231] Fearon K, Strasser F, Anker SD, Bosaeus I, Bruera E, Fainsinger RL, et al. Definition and classification of cancer cachexia: An international consensus. The Lancet Oncology. 2011;**12**(5):489-495

[232] Stolley M, Sheean P, Gerber B, Arroyo C, Schiffer L, Banerjee A, et al. Efficacy of a weight loss intervention for African American breast cancer survivors. Journal of Clinical Oncology. 2017;**35**(24):2820-2828

[233] Colantonio LD, Burrone MS. Factors involved in the paradox of reverse epidemiology. Clinical Nutrition. 2014;**33**(4):729

[234] Banack HR, Kaufman JS. From bad to worse: Collider stratification amplifies confounding bias in the "obesity paradox". European Journal of Epidemiology. 2015;**30**(10):1111-1114

[235] Ligibel JA, Bohlke K, May AM, Clinton SK, Demark-Wahnefried W, Gilchrist SC, et al. Exercise, diet, and weight management during cancer treatment: ASCO guideline. Journal of Clinical Oncology. 2022;**40**(22):2491-2507

Chapter 3

How Increasing Adiposity Impacts Communicable Disease Risk at a Global and a Cellular Level

Andrea Woodcock and Féaron C. Cassidy

Abstract

Obesity is associated with an increased risk of a wide range of morbidities. A major mechanism for this increased risk is dysfunction of the immune system. Immune dysfunction associated with obesity resulting is associated with an increased risk of a number of both communicable and non-communicable diseases. Non-communicable diseases such as type 2 diabetes mellitus (T2DM) make up the majority share of the research and discourse in relation to obesity. However, some infections are found to result in increased disease severity and higher risk of mortality in people with obesity. This was an evident and concerning trend during the severe acute respiratory syndrome coronavirus 2 (SARS-CoV-2) pandemic. Additionally, some vaccines have been found to induce as little as half the protection from disease in people with obesity compared to people without obesity. In this chapter we discuss the impact of obesity during infection and its impact on vaccination—two key considerations that together contribute to the vulnerability of people with obesity, and to public health more generally. We discuss the mechanisms in relation to the dysregulation of immune cells in obesity. Understanding these dysfunctions is crucial and timely as the rates of obesity continue to increase worldwide. Over a billion people worldwide are now living with obesity, resulting in increased individual and population-level disease risk.

Keywords: obesity, immunology, infection, vaccine, immunometabolism, inflammation

1. Introduction

Obesity is an excessive expansion of adipose tissue which can impair an individuals' health [1, 2]. Obesity is chronic and progressive. It is also complex, and multifactorial—involving environmental, genetic, psychological, behavioural, and social factors which affect food preference, food intake, nutrient processing, physical movement behaviours, and cellular metabolic processes [1, 3]. Underweight is also associated with adverse health outcomes, and presents the greater risk for infectious disease compared to obesity. The importance of understanding the impact of obesity on communicable disease risk is emphasised by the increasing prevalence of obesity globally. 6.5% of adults globally are underweight, a number that has been consistently

IntechOpen

falling, while 16.5% of adults globally are living with obesity, and this number is climbing rapidly. There are >1 billion people with obesity worldwide [4].

Obesity is marked by a chronic, low-grade inflammatory state which is intrinsically associated with the host's inflammatory state, frequently termed metabolic inflammation [5, 6]. Inflammation is an immune response, and significant alterations have been reported in the immune system of people with obesity [5]. Obesity promotes dysfunctional metabolic processes via promotion of pro-inflammatory mechanisms, including increased free fatty acids (FFAs), increased reactive oxygen species (ROS) and increased adipocyte stress [7–9].

These alterations contribute to a dysregulation of immune homeostasis within adipose tissue and systemically, resulting in greater levels of pro-inflammatory cytokines, including Tumour Necrosis Factor (TNF)-α and Interleukin (IL)-1 and IL-6 [10, 11]. These inflammatory mediators can exacerbate obesity and increase metabolic dysregulation, underpinning the development of obesity-related diseases. Obesity is commonly associated with an increased risk of developing chronic non-communicable morbidities and diseases including T2DM, cardiovascular disease (CVD) and cancer [9, 12] but is also a risk factor for infectious disease. Obesity has also been associated with impaired vaccine responses, thereby further increasing infection risk, with potential public health implications.

The initial trigger of inflammation remains unclear but is connected to adipose tissue dysfunction. Adipose tissue expansion is characteristic of obesity. Adipose is not merely an energy store, but also functions as an endocrine organ, producing cytokines (termed adipokines) which impact metabolism through the enhancing or dampening of inflammation [11]. The loss of adipose tissue homeostasis, including changes to adipose-resident immune cells, plays an important role in the systemic inflammation observed in people with obesity (**Figure 1**).

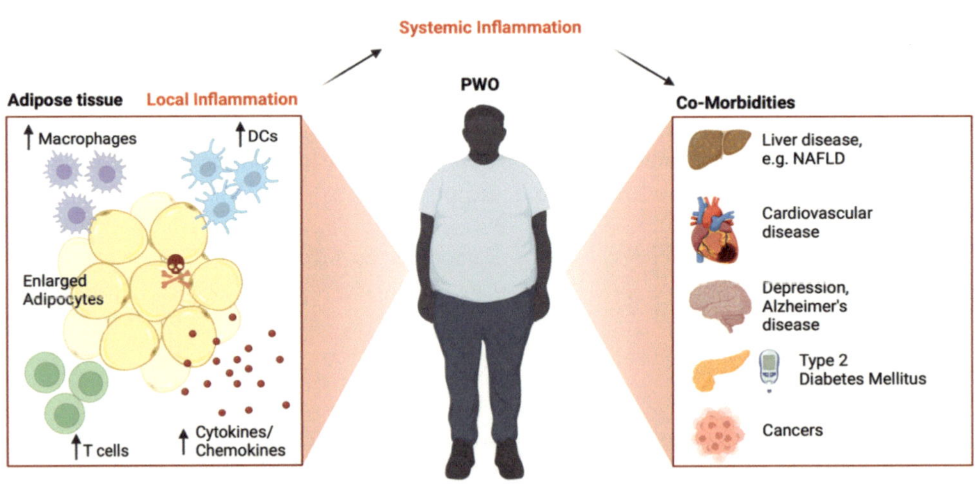

Figure 1.
Impact of obesity on adipose tissue driving local and systemic inflammation and associated co-morbidities. Obesity can induce adipocyte hypertrophy and adipocyte cell death which can recruit immune cells with pro-inflammatory properties (e.g., macrophages/dendritic cells/T cells). Adipocytes secrete chemokines and cytokines (e.g., MCP-1, TNF-α, IL-6) which promote immune cell infiltration and activation respectively. Local inflammation can spread inducing the chronic, low-grade inflammation observed in obesity, which is linked to an increased risk of multiple co-morbidities (e.g., non-alcoholic fatty liver disease (NAFLD), cancers, depression) (adapted from Barakat and Almeida [13]; Lim and Boster [14]). Created in BioRender. Woodcock, A. & Hogan, A. (2025) https://BioRender.com/sn58poo.

Chronic inflammation can drive insulin resistance in its target organs, resulting in greater insulin production by the pancreas [15]. Ultimately, the resistance to insulin can induce a hyperglycaemic state due to the inability of host tissues to take up glucose and normalise blood glucose levels, marking the onset of T2DM [15]. Hyperlipidaemia, another characteristic of obesity, can lead to plaque formation within blood vessels and the heart, resulting in hypertension and CVD [16]. This systemic dysfunction is associated with production of pro-inflammatory cytokines and increased levels of pro-inflammatory cells [5]. Both innate and adaptive cell populations can be affected in obesity to favour a pro-inflammatory state, alongside a decline in inflammation resolution pathways [17]. People with obesity may generate suboptimal or inadequate responses following infection or vaccination rendering them more susceptible to adverse effects when exposed to pathogens [18, 19]. Epidemiologically, people with obesity are found to be at greater risk of acquiring infection and of increased infection severity [20, 21].

Children with obesity are at 80% risk of having obesity in adulthood [22], and defects in metabolism, hormones, and cells, can persist after weight loss [23, 24] even driving regaining of weight [25]. The most effective treatments for people with obesity are invasive bariatric surgery and low-availability glucagon-like peptide-1 (GLP1)-receptor agonists (RAs) [26–28]. These GLP-1 RAs mimic naturally occurring GLP-1 and act to induce satiety, slow gastric emptying, and induce insulin secretion [29]. Initially approved for the treatment of T2DM, weight loss was observed in these individuals and since 2014 these drugs have been approved to treat obesity [30]. Despite global public health efforts, obesity is a health concern set to continue increasing in prevalence, associated with serious unmet clinical needs on an individual and population level. Though often overlooked, the interaction between obesity and infectious disease risk is an important consideration for public health planning.

2. The immune system in obesity

Immune cell number and function can both be altered in obesity. Similar to ageing [31], obesity causes skewing of haematopoiesis towards a myeloid lineage [32] and can result in a reduction in lymphoid subsets [33]. Oxidative stress has been shown to cause dysfunction in the bone marrow [34]. Its subsequent impact on the various cell subsets within the bone marrow and those which egress requires further elucidation. Functionally, immune cells can be impeded by the obese micro environmental conditions. In the resting state, immune cells exhibit a low basal metabolism but upon activation they become highly metabolically active utilising a significant portion of the body's energy [35, 36]. This fuels the downstream activities of the activated immune cell, including protein synthesis, and the effectiveness of these downstream functions is tied to nutrient availability [37, 38]. The increase of FFAs in obesity can impact cell function [39]. FFA can induce ROS production, in turn, promoting endoplasmic reticulum (ER) stress and increased adipose tissue expression of pro-inflammatory genes [40–42]. Obesity impacts immune cell metabolism and in turn their function. It can change intrinsic cellular metabolic pathways, e.g. favouring mitochondrial respiration ultimately increasing ROS and impeding their effector function [43].

2.1 Innate immunity in obesity

One of the defining factors of obesity-associated chronic inflammation is the localisation of myeloid cells to organs involved in metabolism, including the white adipose tissue [44]. Chemokines, such as RANTES (*r*egulated on *a*ctivation, *n*ormal *T*-cell *e*xpressed and *s*ecreted), have higher expression levels in the adipose tissue of diet-induced obesity in mice or people with obesity, influencing cell migration and accumulation [45–47]. Increased uptake of lipids within adipose tissue results in both hypertrophy and hyperplasia of adipocytes [11]. Enlarged adipocytes can upregulate stress signals, signalling to the immune system for action, resulting in an inflammatory response [48, 49]. Unchecked these enlarged adipocytes can become necrotic, initiating a high-inflammatory state [50]. Inflammation, hyperplasia and limited oxygen availability can produce a hypoxic environment within adipose tissue [11]. Elevated levels of Hypoxia-Inducible Factor (HIF)-1α have been reported in obesity [51]. A hypoxic environment can trigger adipocyte death, promoting infiltration of macrophages and free FFA release into the blood [11, 52]. Lipid circulation can lead to its deposition in other non-adipose tissues, e.g. liver and muscle. FFA can activate toll-like receptors (TLRs), TLR4 in particular, and downstream signalling results in the production of cytokines [53]. Elevated expression of monocyte chemoattractant protein (MCP-1), IL-6 and TNF-α is associated with increased adipocyte death [54]. MCP-1 is also known as C−C motif chemokine ligand (CCL) 2 [55]. MCP-1 attracts monocytes, including macrophages, to the site of inflammation, the adipose tissue [54, 55]. The pro-inflammatory cytokines, TNF-α and IL-6, can promote exacerbation of inflammation from local to systemic [11].

In addition to the systemic inflammation, obesity can affect both innate and adaptive immune cell populations, importantly those involved in host-pathogen defences [39, 56, 57]. A source of pro-inflammatory cytokines, IL-1β and IL-18, was traced back to macrophages in high fat diet mice. These cells contained high concentrations of palmitate, a saturated fatty acid, which activated the inflammasome and subsequently the production of these cytokines [58]. *Macrophages* with a pro-inflammatory M1-like polarisation, rather than the anti-inflammatory M2-like state are observed in adipose tissue in mice fed a high fat diet [48]. As macrophages constitute a large proportion of the leukocyte population in the adipose tissue [59], dysregulation of these cells can result in subsequent alteration in their function of maintaining adipose tissue homeostasis. Macrophage numbers increase with increasing adipose tissue mass, observed upon high fat diet feeding [60, 61]. The production of chemokines from adipose tissue macrophages can recruit other immune cells, including monocytes [62], which exacerbates inflammation within the adipose tissue.

Natural Killer (*NK*) cells are an important innate effector population with potent anti-viral activities. NK cells can detect virally infected cells and function by releasing cytotoxic granules capable of killing these infected cells [63]. People with obesity display reduced NK cell activity, observed through defective effector molecule production and cytotoxicity, which can commence early during childhood [39, 64–66]. Reduced NK cell cytotoxicity was observed in the lung and spleen of influenza-infected high fat diet mice compared to low fat diet [67]. Lipid accumulation, due to obesity, has been shown to impede NK cell function, including decreased interferon (IFN)-γ production [39]. Interferons are essential anti-viral cytokines [68]. The inability of these key innate cells to function within people with obesity may be correlated with increased susceptibility to viral infections [20, 21].

Another innate lymphocyte population, Mucosal associated invariant T (*MAIT*) cells which have important effector functions, has been found to contribute to chronic inflammation via an IL-17 producing phenotype in obesity [57, 69, 70]. The unrestrained production of this cytokine can have detrimental consequences [69, 71, 72]. MAIT cells upon activation increase their rates of glycolysis to support their effector functions [73]. However, in people with obesity, MAIT cells were shown to have reduced levels of glycolysis, following activation, compared to healthy control donors without obesity [73]. Decreased glycolytic rates impacted MAIT cell function, observed via a reduction in IFN-γ producing MAIT cells in people with obesity [73]. The reduction in glycolysis was due to defective mammalian target of rapamycin complex (mTORC) 1 (described as a master regulator of metabolism), demonstrated by a reduction in phosphorylation of ribosomal protein S6 (a target of mTORC1) [73], and defects in MYC, another metabolic regulator [74].

Neutrophils are the most abundant circulating leukocyte and are the first responders during infection or inflammation. Neutrophils have also been observed to be increased in the circulation of children and adults living with obesity [75, 76]. Transient adipose tissue infiltration by neutrophils has been observed early during high fat diet feeding of mice [77]. More recently, enzymes involved in ROS production, such as myeloperoxidase (MPO) or inducible nitric oxide synthase (iNOS), were increased in expression or activity respectively, in bone marrow-derived neutrophils from mice on a high fat diet [78]. McDowell et al. [78] found that the increased neutrophil ROS activity weakened vascular integrity and promoted greater tumour metastasis in the mice on the high fat diet compared to low fat diet. Increased circulating MPO has been observed in people with severe obesity (average body mass index (BMI) >40 kg/m^2) compared to controls, along with increased expression of activation marker, CD66b, on neutrophils [79]. Obesity can result in the dysfunction of different innate immune cells which can perpetuate the inflammatory state. However, their dysfunction also has implications for host responses against pathogens, cancer or vaccinations. Immune cell dysregulation can also be observed in adaptive immune subsets.

2.2 Innate-adaptive crosstalk in obesity

Dendritic cells (DCs) are phagocytic, innate immune cells which act as professional antigen presenting cells to activate the adaptive immune response [80, 81]. DCs circulate the body in an immature state, upon antigen encounter, DCs undergo maturation [80]. Immature DCs have a high phagocytic capacity, sampling antigen in their surroundings [82–84]. Upon maturation, their phagocytic machinery is downregulated and DCs upregulate the expression of molecules required for antigen presentation [84]. DCs express major histocompatibility complexes (MHCs) to present antigen and co-stimulatory molecules which provide additional signals for efficient T cell activation [84]. DCs also produce cytokines which can polarise T cell differentiation and enhance the activation of other immune cells [85, 86]. In these ways, dendritic cells bridge the innate and adaptive immune systems.

Numerous alterations to DC function have been described in the context of obesity. Interestingly, increased numbers of DCs and their increased expression of activation and maturation markers and loss of homeostatic, anti-inflammatory profile was specific to metabolic organs including adipose tissue, with the peripheral blood exhibiting a decrease in both [87–90].

Similarly to innate lymphocytes, despite the chronic inflammatory state in obesity, acute DC responses to infection are muted, and even anti-inflammatory in people with obesity [43, 89]. This is exacerbated by modified chemokine (including increased C-C chemokine receptor 7 (CCR7), a marker of migratory capacity) and co-stimulatory molecule expression profiles [91, 92]. That these changes are mediated by DC metabolism is indicated by the increase in fatty acid oxidation and therefore mitochondrial respiration and ROS observed after high fat diet in mice [43, 93]. The reduced number and infection-response function of dendritic cells results in impaired T lymphocyte activation, proliferation and differentiation in people with obesity, with implications for infection and vaccination [87, 88, 94–99].

2.3 Adaptive immunity in obesity

In adipose tissue, in the context of obesity, pro-inflammatory $CD8^+$ T and $CD4^+$ T helper (Th) 1 and Th17 cells are favoured and accumulate while there is a loss of anti-inflammatory $CD4^+$ Th2 and regulatory T cells (Treg) [11, 100, 101]. Favouring of Th1 or Th17 effector T cell differentiation promotes the inflammatory state [87, 102, 103]. The Th2 cytokine, IL-4, was increased in T cell co-cultures with dendritic cells from people with obesity compared to control dendritic cells [89]. Skewing towards an immunosuppressive state would impede the effective clearance of infected cells and pathogens.

Sheridan et al. [94] studied the effect of BMI on adaptive immune responses in humans following influenza vaccination. People with obesity had a decrease in percentage of influenza-activated $CD8^+$ T cells and a significant decrease in activity compared to controls [94], their activity measured via the proportion of cells expressing Granzyme B and IFN-γ. Hence these $CD8^+$ T cells were less capable of lysing infected cells and inhibiting viral replication [104, 105]. Further murine work observed an impairment in memory T cell responses to influenza, underpinned by alterations in T cell metabolism due to obesity [106]. Importantly, this impairment of memory T cells and their associated metabolic dysfunction was not reversed following weight loss [106].

The addition of antioxidants has previously been shown to improve T cell proliferation and reduce oxidative stress [107]. ROS accumulation causes immune dysfunction, e.g., preventing the proliferation of T cells and inducing apoptosis instead [108]. Saturated fatty acids can be detected by TLR4 on the surface of innate cells, which contributes to the pro-inflammatory state due to the production of pro-inflammatory cytokines downstream [53, 109]. The production and secretion of the cytokine TNF has been well-documented in its ability to impair insulin sensitivity and glucose metabolism and contribute to insulin resistance within the host [110]. mTORC1 is a master regulator of cellular metabolism [38]. Its key role is to sense nutrients, growth factors and the energy status of the cell and functions accordingly [38, 111, 112].

There are different types of T cells including Tregs which serve homeostatic roles, e.g. inflammation resolution and tissue repair, and are detected by their expression of the master regulator FoxP3 [113]. Tregs were significantly decreased in visceral or abdominal fat of high fat diet mice compared to controls [113, 114]. Deiuliis et al. [113] discovered reduced FOXP3 in the visceral adipose tissue of people with obesity. Wagner et al. [115] expanded on these studies and found decreased Tregs in circulation of people with obesity compared to controls. Reduced Tregs was predictive of higher markers of inflammation (measured via plasma C-reactive protein) in circulation [115]. A decrease in Tregs can perturb normal host immune homeostasis, possibly contributing to the dysregulated inflammatory state. γδ T cells are an unconventional group of T cells involved in pathogen clearance and tissue homeostasis, Vγ9Vδ2 T cells comprise the largest group of γδ T cells, with crucial anti-viral function [116]. Reduced circulating Vγ9Vδ2 T cells were observed in people with obesity compared to controls, these cells also displayed impaired IFN-γ production following influenza stimulation [116]. Overall, these studies display a myriad of obesity-associated impacts on the T cell arm of the adaptive immune response. The inability of these cells to respond effectively to particularly viral stimulation may contribute to the increased susceptibility and morbidity to viral infection in people with obesity, described further in Section 3.1.

B cells form the humoral response of adaptive immunity. People with obesity have been reported in some but not all studies to have an increased frequency of naïve B cells [117, 118]. Wijngaarden et al. [118] postulated that B cells exit the bone marrow and enter the blood and tissues due the chronic inflammatory state. Šlisere et al. [119] elaborated on these different B cell subsets in circulation of people with obesity to show a trending increase in mature B cells and a significant decrease in total memory B cells compared to controls. The impact of obesity on memory B cell populations has negative implications for vaccination strategies or re-exposure to a pathogen, where the humoral immune response may be slower due to lower memory populations. Interestingly, bariatric surgery restored all these B cell subset changes in people with obesity to resemble the controls [119]—a positive observation for the treatment of obesity.

3. The impact of obesity on infectious diseases

The inflammatory state observed in obesity, as well as its comorbidities, can increase susceptibility, morbidity and mortality to infections [9]. Infections including Human Immunodeficiency Virus (HIV), tuberculosis, malaria and hepatitis are responsible for high morbidity burdens globally, but their prevalence and impact are concentrated in lower income countries [120–125]. The proportion of deaths in 2015 due to infectious disease across all age groups in low income countries was approximately 30% while in high income countries it was approximately 8% [124]. The pattern for obesity prevalence is opposite—low income countries with the highest risk from communicable diseases tend to be those with lower BMIs, while high income countries have the lowest risk of communicable disease and the highest rates of obesity – for example many countries in sub-Saharan Africa have some of the lowest rates of obesity and the highest burden of infectious disease, while countries in North America record the opposite pattern (**Figure 2**) [4]. This pattern has contributed to a paucity of data on the co-occurrence of obesity and major global infectious diseases, but the recent SARS-CoV-2 pandemic highlighted the importance of increasing our understanding in this area [21]. During the coronavirus disease 2019 (COVID-19) pandemic there was a greater risk of severe disease and death recorded in people with obesity compared to matched controls without obesity [21].

The rates of obesity are increasing in all geographic regions, including in sub-Saharan Africa [4]. Concomitantly, there is increasing risk from novel infectious diseases globally due to the recorded increasing rates of antimicrobial resistance, as well as climate change [126, 127]. Taken together, these trends indicate that the current broad mutual exclusivity of high infectious disease burden and obesity will not continue, and that there is a clinical and public health incentive for increased understanding of their coexistence.

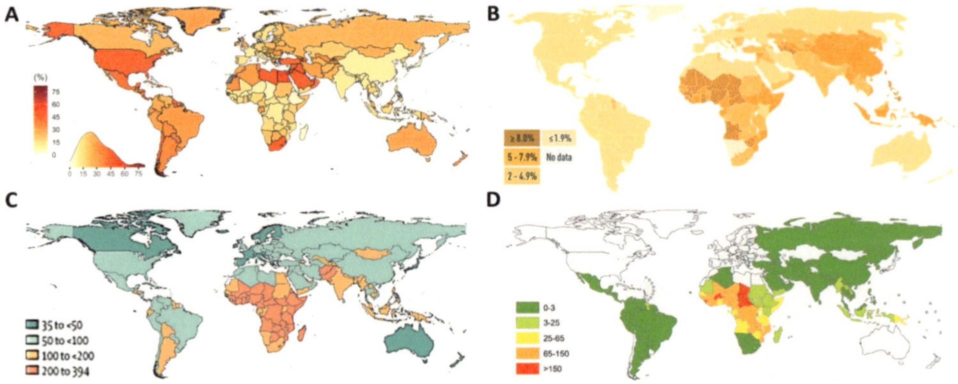

Figure 2.
A general global trend for coincidence of high rates of infectious diseases and lower rates of obesity, and vice versa. (A) Age-standardised prevalence of obesity in 2022; directly from supplementary materials of NCD Risk Factor Collaboration study published 2024 [4], (B) Countries most affected by hepatitis B, image modified from the Hepatitis B CDC Yellow Book 2024 [120], (C) Overall age-standardised mortality rate per 100,000 population for 33 bacterial pathogens responsible for >55% of infection-related deaths globally; image modified from that created by the GBD (Global Burden of Disease) 2019 Antimicrobial Resistance Collaborators [121], (D) Global malaria death rates 2012; image modified from Poostchi et al. [122].

3.1 Viral infection in obesity

Risk of disease and mortality are associated with underweight but not obesity in relation to HIV infection [128, 129]. In contrast, severity of liver disease in Hepatitis C infection, and risk of developing hepatocellular carcinoma in Hepatitis B infection are both increased in association with obesity [130, 131]. Non-alcoholic fatty liver disease (NAFLD), which has increased globally in association with obesity, is found at higher rates in people with obesity and the dual presence of hepatitis and NAFLD likely explains the observed increased severity [131–133].

Respiratory tract infections, most commonly caused by viruses, are more common in and result in higher symptom burden in people with obesity [134]. Higher BMI has been found to correlate with acute respiratory infection susceptibility in children, with risk of infection in overweight children double that of those of a lower BMI [135]. Further evidence for excess susceptibility to viral infection in people with obesity comes from the influenza A H1N1 pandemic (H1N1pdm) which occurred in 2009–2010 [20]. Data from approximately 70,000 hospitalised H1N1-positive patients across 19 countries or administrative regions were examined to identify influenza-associated risk factors [20]. Risk factors were classified into hospitalisation, ICU admission and fatality, based on infection severity. The findings revealed a positive correlation between infection severity and the proportion of H1N1-positive patients having at least one chronic condition. Chronic conditions, e.g. pulmonary disease, diabetes or CVD, and immunodeficiency were determined to be risk factors for severe H1N1pdm infection, similar to seasonal influenza [20, 136]. However, morbid obesity was then recognised as a risk factor for severe influenza infection [20]. Disease severity correlated with an increasing percentage of patients with obesity (BMI ≥30 kg/m^2), with a similar trend in patients with a BMI >40 kg/m^2, classified as morbid obesity. Patients with obesity or morbid obesity have a greater risk of ICU admission [137, 138], but there are associated complications, where these same individuals have been reported to have an increased susceptibility to nosocomial or secondary infections [139]. As a result, people with obesity face additional risks of contracting secondary microbial infections, when hospitalised, such as catheter-related infections or ventilator-associated pneumonia. These substantially elevate their mortality risk.

Following the H1N1 pandemic, the Middle East respiratory syndrome coronavirus (MERS-CoV) surfaced in 2012, with a high mortality rate, especially in patients with comorbidities. A meta-analysis of MERS-CoV cases observed 16% of the cases occurred in people with obesity [140]. During the COVID-19 pandemic caused by SARS-CoV-2, it became apparent that obesity greatly increased the risk of COVID-19 infection, over 46% increased risk. A meta-analysis found that people with obesity were more likely to be hospitalised (113% increased risk), admitted to intensive care unit (ICU) (74%) and die (48%) due to COVID-19 [21]. Impaired responses to infection in people with obesity raise concerns whether an adequate memory response is generated following infection.

3.2 Bacterial and parasitic infection in obesity

Unlike viral infections, the relationship between obesity and other infections is less clear due to a paucity of data, partly attributable to the aforementioned epidemiology of both (**Figure 2**). Urinary tract, surgical site and bloodstream infection risk have been found to have increased incidence in people with obesity, especially in patients with morbid obesity and in those with excess adiposity [141–143]. In the case of both urinary tract and surgical site infections there is a lack of clarity on the topic due to sometimes opposite findings most likely due to the U-shaped curve whereby adverse outcomes also associate with underweight, and due to confounding variables [141, 144–146]. For example, risk of sepsis-related mortality is higher in both those with BMI <20 and those with BMI above 30 [147]. Streptococcus and pneumococcus infection, as well as colonisation with staphylococcus (recorded as an indicator of subsequent infection risk) were all higher in people with obesity compared to those without obesity and above the underweight threshold [148–152]. Though not all studies assessed underweight, when assessed, underweight also correlates with worse outcomes. Tuberculosis in particular has a demonstratable association with underweight, and a relationship with BMI that places overweight and obesity favourably in terms of outcome [153–156]. However, there is a dearth of studies that included participants with a BMI over 30. Therefore, it is unclear if more severely high BMI would be associated with poorer outcomes as per other bacterial infectious diseases, or afford the same protections as an overweight BMI has been shown to do. Similarly to the overall pattern observed in bacterial infections, increased severity of malaria is associated with both extremes of BMI [157–159].

4. The impact of obesity on vaccination

Successful vaccination strategies depend on the stimulation of both arms of the immune response, innate and adaptive [160]. However, challenges occur when underlying conditions cause immune dysregulation, such as obesity [94, 101]. Obesity results in immune dysfunction through various mechanisms, affecting the responses necessary for effective vaccination: the innate, humoral and T-cell mediated immune responses [24, 89, 106]. Accumulating evidence in people with obesity highlights their diminished ability to elicit optimal immune responses compared to controls following vaccination [94]. Immune memory responses develop following vaccination and serve to protect the inoculated host upon exposure to the causative pathogen [160]. Using influenza viruses as an example, the activation of T-cell responses is particularly important due to their targeting of internal proteins that are often conserved amongst viral strains [161]. Humoral antibody (Ab)-based responses target surface proteins which can differ between viral strains [162]. Studies in mice with diet-induced obesity by Karlsson et al. [101] found a significant reduction in memory T cell function, specific for influenza, in mice with diet-induced obesity-compared to controls. A subsequent study showed a decrease in the maintenance of these influenza-specific $CD8^+$ memory T cells in the mice with diet-induced obesity [163].

The ability to confer protection upon secondary infection correlates with the number of these specific memory T cells within the target tissue [163], in this context, the lungs. Two cytokines have displayed important regulatory roles in antigen (Ag)-specific $CD8^+$ memory T cell maintenance, IL-7 and IL-15 [163]. Karlsson et al. [163] hypothesised the following mechanisms as explanations for their observations. Hyperleptinaemia is a characteristic of obesity which can lead to resistance to leptin [164]; leptin is a hormone shown to link metabolism and the immune system [165]. Karlsson et al. [163] observed diminished bystander memory T cell proliferation over time in high fat diet mice, despite higher *Il15* mRNA expression. The impairment of leptin signalling was given as a possible explanation for the reduction in memory T cell numbers, as leptin signalling has been associated with IL-15 function [163]. Dysregulation of leptin and leptin receptor signalling has been associated with higher risk of infection in both insufficient and excess adiposity [166]. As previously mentioned, obesity can affect antigen-presenting cell function, importantly dendritic cells [89] which are required for memory T cell maintenance via trans-presentation of IL-15 on its respective receptor [167]. Hence, obesity can impede the activation of a rapid immune response upon exposure to the specific antigen in vaccinated individuals through its reduction in number and function of these vital memory T cells. These results have broader public health implications as weight loss may not adequately reverse certain immune dysfunction [23, 106], unlike its reversal of certain associated comorbidities [168], therefore, maintaining diminished vaccine efficacy and infection susceptibility in people with obesity.

A year after vaccination, individuals with a higher BMI had a significant reduction in influenza-specific antibody titres [94]. People with obesity following receipt of the Hepatitis B virus (HBV) vaccine had significantly less Abs compared to controls [19, 169]. Non-responsiveness to the HBV vaccine correlated with increasing BMI [169]. Obesity can also hinder vaccination efficacy against other pathogens, e.g. bacteria, where over-weight children, compared to controls, showed a significant reduction in anti-tetanus antibody levels [170]. As a result, obesity would cause greater susceptibility to these viruses or bacteria, in turn, affecting infection severity.

During the COVID-19 pandemic, various studies were performed to investigate the effect of SARS-CoV-2 on the humoral and cell-mediated response pre- and post-vaccination. Pre-vaccination people with obesity had greater neutralising antibody and spike-specific IgG titres which was proposed to be due to a more overreactive immune response which is disadvantageous during infection [171]. Similar levels of circulating T cells specific for SARS-CoV-2 spike and membrane peptides were detected in people with obesity who survived infection compared to controls [172]. However, higher frequencies were detected in a different study 12 months after infection [171] which was inferred to possibly explain the finding that increased BMI correlated with an increased risk of long COVID [173]. A meta-analysis determined reduced antibody responses following SARS-CoV-2 vaccination of people with obesity [174]. Onyango et al. [171] demonstrated a decreasing trend in neutralising to spike IgG titre ratio for people with obesity compared to controls after infection and vaccination. However, it was shown that vaccination did boost both cellular and humoral responses similarly between people with obesity, overweight and control individuals [171]. SARS-CoV-2 spike specific T cells, including polyfunctional T cells, were comparable between people with obesity and controls following ChAdOx1 COVID-19 vaccination [175]. Evidence still shows that obesity is a risk factor for infection and vaccination, however, data where vaccination yields comparable cell-mediated immune responses is positive for people living with obesity.

Various mechanisms may influence vaccine efficacy in people with obesity. Firstly, immune dysfunction can result in suboptimal vaccine responses, where people with obesity may not generate an adequate immune response upon inoculation (including a memory response), hence diminishing the protection upon future antigen exposure. Secondly, drug pharmacokinetics must be considered, as greater body mass (associated with obesity) may affect the uptake, absorption and distribution of vaccines in people with obesity after inoculation [170]. These factors require consideration during vaccine development to ensure the desired immune response is not compromised. As research has shown that, despite vaccination, adults living with obesity compared to vaccinated controls, were twice at risk of developing influenza or influenza-like infections [176] demonstrating people with obesity as an at-risk group for increased susceptibility to infection and greater infection morbidity and mortality [20, 21].

Understanding the causes and consequences of obesity is crucial for improving human health. While preventative measures remain the most optimal strategy for mitigating disease, the global surge in cases of obesity over the past 40 years [2], underlines the need for effective treatment to combat this condition.

5. Conclusion

Obesity is a chronic and multifactorial disease, associated with over 200 chronic comorbidities [2, 12], including an increased susceptibility, morbidity, and mortality to infection [20, 21]. Multiple genetic and environmental factors influence the development and progression of obesity [1, 177]. People with obesity may experience a decreased quality of life and reduced life expectancy [178, 179]. The disease exerts profound mental, emotional and physical tolls on the affected individuals and greater understanding is required to address its associated vulnerabilities, as any dysfunction may not be reversed following weight loss [23, 24, 106]. People with obesity may have impaired infection clearance or more frequent infections due to a suboptimal immune system, alongside potentially associated chronic illnesses [180]. The effects of obesity on immune cell compartments are clear [57, 64, 89, 94], fortunately pharmaceutical treatments are showing NK cell improvements [23] and further elucidation of these treatments on other immune cells is required. Altogether, these data reiterate the need for concerted public health strategies to address rising obesity rates, as the disease continues to have detrimental economic and social effects across the globe [3].

Author details

Andrea Woodcock[1] and Féaron C. Cassidy[2,3*]

1 School of Biochemistry and Immunology, Trinity Biomedical Sciences Institute, Trinity College Dublin, Dublin, Ireland

2 Kathleen Lonsdale Institute for Human Health Research, Maynooth University, Maynooth, Co Kildare, Ireland

3 Department of Medicine Huddinge, Center for Infectious Medicine, Karolinska Institutet, Karolinska, Sweden

*Address all correspondence to: fearon.cassidy@mu.ie

IntechOpen

© 2025 The Author(s). Licensee IntechOpen. This chapter is distributed under the terms of the Creative Commons Attribution License (http://creativecommons.org/licenses/by/3.0), which permits unrestricted use, distribution, and reproduction in any medium, provided the original work is properly cited.

References

[1] Bray GA, Kim KK, JPH W, Federation on behalf of the WO. Obesity: A chronic relapsing progressive disease process. A position statement of the world obesity federation. Obesity Reviews. 2017;**18**(7):715-723

[2] WHO. Obesity and Overweight. Geneva, Switzerland: WHO; 2024. Available from: https://www.who.int/news-room/fact-sheets/detail/obesity-and-overweight [Accessed: February 12, 2025]

[3] Anekwe CV, Jarrell AR, Townsend MJ, Gaudier GI, Hiserodt JM, Stanford FC. Socioeconomics of obesity. Current Obesity Reports. 2020;**9**(3):272-279

[4] Collaboration (NCD-RisC) NRF, Salmerón Martínez D. Worldwide trends in underweight and obesity from 1990 to 2022: A pooled analysis of 3663 population representative studies with 222 million children, adolescents, and adults. The Lancet. 2024;**403**:1027-1050

[5] Fantuzzi G. Adipose tissue, adipokines, and inflammation. Journal of Allergy and Clinical Immunology. 2005;**115**(5):911-919

[6] Xu H. Obesity and metabolic inflammation. Drug Discovery Today: Disease Mechanisms. 2013;**10**(1):e21-e25

[7] Wolowczuk I, Verwaerde C, Viltart O, Delanoye A, Delacre M, Pot B, et al. Feeding our immune system: Impact on metabolism. Journal of Immunology Research. 2008;**2008**(1). Available from: https://onlinelibrary.wiley.com/doi/epdf/10.1155/2008/639803

[8] Minihane AM, Vinoy S, Russell WR, Baka A, Roche HM, Tuohy KM, et al. Low-grade inflammation, diet composition and health: Current research evidence and its translation. The British Journal of Nutrition. 2015;**114**(7):999-1012

[9] Haslam DW, James WPT. Obesity. The Lancet. 2005;**366**(9492):1197-1209

[10] Trayhurn P, Wood IS. Adipokines: Inflammation and the pleiotropic role of white adipose tissue. The British Journal of Nutrition. 2004;**92**(3):347-355

[11] Chan PC, Hsieh PS. The role of adipocyte hypertrophy and hypoxia in the development of obesity-associated adipose tissue inflammation and insulin resistance. Adiposity - Omics and Molecular Understanding. 2017;**10**:127-141

[12] Horn DB, Almandoz JP, Look M. What is clinically relevant weight loss for your patients and how can it be achieved? A narrative review. Postgraduate Medicine. 2022;**134**(4):359-375

[13] Barakat B, Almeida MEF. Biochemical and immunological changes in obesity. Archives of Biochemistry and Biophysics. 2021;**708**:108951

[14] Lim Y, Boster J. Obesity and Comorbid Conditions. Treasure Island (FL): StatPearls Publishing; 2024. Available from: http://www.ncbi.nlm.nih.gov/books/NBK574535/

[15] Bazotte RB, Silva LG, Schiavon FPM. Insulin resistance in the liver: Deficiency or excess of insulin? Cell Cycle. 2014;**13**(16):2494-2494

[16] Jung UJ, Choi MS. Obesity and its metabolic complications: The role of Adipokines and the relationship between obesity, inflammation, insulin resistance,

dyslipidemia and nonalcoholic fatty liver disease. International Journal of Molecular Sciences. 2014;**15**(4):6184-6223

[17] Luo B, Wang Z, Zhang Z, Shen Z, Zhang Z. The deficiency of macrophage erythropoietin signaling contributes to delayed acute inflammation resolution in diet-induced obese mice. Biochimica et Biophysica Acta (BBA) - Molecular Basis of Disease. 2019;**1865**(2):339-349

[18] Banga N, Guss P, Banga A, Rosenman KD. Incidence and variables associated with inadequate antibody titers after pre-exposure rabies vaccination among veterinary medical students. Vaccine. 2014;**32**(8):979-983

[19] Mckee CM, Mcevoy MB, Duke P, Kelsey MC. Effectiveness of intradermal hepatitis B immunization of hospital staff. International Journal of STD and AIDS. 1990;**1**(1):32-34

[20] Van Kerkhove MD, Vandemaele KAH, Shinde V, Jaramillo-Gutierrez G, Koukounari A, Donnelly CA, et al. Risk factors for severe outcomes following 2009 influenza a (H1N1) infection: A global pooled analysis. PLoS Medicine. 2011;**8**(7):e1001053

[21] Popkin BM, Du S, Green WD, Beck MA, Algaith T, Herbst CH, et al. Individuals with obesity and COVID-19: A global perspective on the epidemiology and biological relationships. Obesity Reviews. 2020;**21**(11):e13128

[22] Simmonds M, Llewellyn A, Owen CG, Woolacott N. Predicting adult obesity from childhood obesity: A systematic review and meta-analysis. Obesity Reviews. 2016;**17**(2):95-107

[23] De Barra C, Khalil M, Mat A, O'Donnell C, Shaamile F, Brennan K, et al. Glucagon-like peptide-1 therapy in people with obesity restores natural killer cell metabolism and effector function. Obesity. 2023;**31**(7):1787-1797

[24] Frasca D, Romero M, Diaz A, Blomberg BB. Obesity accelerates age defects in B cells, and weight loss improves B cell function. Immunity & Ageing. 2023;**20**(1):35

[25] Vink RG, Roumans NJT, Arkenbosch LAJ, Mariman ECM, Van Baak MA. The effect of rate of weight loss on long-term weight regain in adults with overweight and obesity. Obesity. 2016;**24**(2):321-327

[26] Wolfe BM, Kvach E, Eckel RH. Treatment of obesity: Weight loss and bariatric surgery. Circulation Research. 2016;**118**(11):1844-1844

[27] Sjöström L, Peltonen M, Jacobson P, Sjöström CD, Karason K, Wedel H, et al. Bariatric surgery and long-term cardiovascular events. Journal of the American Medical Association. 2012;**307**(1):56-65

[28] Chakhtoura M, Haber R, Ghezzawi M, Rhayem C, Tcheroyan R, Mantzoros CS. Pharmacotherapy of obesity: An update on the available medications and drugs under investigation. eClinicalMedicine. 2023;**58**:101882. Available from: https://www.sciencedirect.com/science/article/pii/S2589537023000597?via%3Dihub

[29] Flint A, Raben A, Astrup A, Holst JJ. Glucagon-like peptide 1 promotes satiety and suppresses energy intake in humans. The Journal of Clinical Investigation. 1998;**101**(3):515-520

[30] Drucker DJ. Efficacy and safety of GLP-1 medicines for type 2 diabetes and obesity. Diabetes Care. 2024;**47**(11):1873-1888

[31] Pang WW, Price EA, Sahoo D, Beerman I, Maloney WJ, Rossi DJ, et al. Human bone marrow hematopoietic stem cells are increased in frequency and myeloid-biased with age. Proceedings of the National Academy of Sciences of the United States of America. 2011;**108**(50):20012-20017

[32] Nagareddy PR, Kraakman M, Masters SL, Stirzaker RA, Gorman DJ, Grant RW, et al. Adipose tissue macrophages promote myelopoiesis and monocytosis in obesity. Cell Metabolism. 2014;**19**(5):821-835

[33] Adler BJ, Green DE, Pagnotti GM, Chan ME, Rubin CT. High fat diet rapidly suppresses B Lymphopoiesis by disrupting the supportive capacity of the bone marrow niche. PLoS One. 2014;**9**(3):e90639

[34] Lee JM, Govindarajah V, Goddard B, Hinge A, Muench DE, Filippi MD, et al. Obesity alters the long-term fitness of the hematopoietic stem cell compartment through modulation of Gfi1 expression. The Journal of Experimental Medicine. 2018;**215**(2):627-644

[35] Ganeshan K, Nikkanen J, Man K, Leong YA, Sogawa Y, Maschek JA, et al. Energetic trade-offs and Hypometabolic states promote disease tolerance. Cell. 2019;**177**(2):399-413

[36] Almajwal A, Alam I, Zeb F, Fatima S, Almajwal A, Alam I, et al. Energy metabolism and allocation in selfish immune system and brain: A beneficial role of insulin resistance in aging. Food and Nutrition Sciences. 2018;**10**(1):64-80

[37] Krawczyk CM, Holowka T, Sun J, Blagih J, Amiel E, DeBerardinis RJ, et al. Toll-like receptor–induced changes in glycolytic metabolism regulate dendritic cell activation. Blood. 2010;**115**(23):4742-4749

[38] O'Neill LAJ, Kishton RJ, Rathmell J. A guide to immunometabolism for immunologists. Nature Reviews Immunology. 2016;**16**(9):553-565

[39] Michelet X, Dyck L, Hogan A, Loftus RM, Duquette D, Wei K, et al. Metabolic reprogramming of natural killer cells in obesity limits antitumor responses. Nature Immunology. 2018;**19**(12):1330-1340

[40] Erbay E, Babaev VR, Mayers JR, Makowski L, Charles KN, Snitow ME, et al. Reducing endoplasmic reticulum stress through a macrophage lipid chaperone alleviates atherosclerosis. Nature Medicine. 2009;**15**(12):1383-1391

[41] Savva C, Copson E, Johnson PWM, Cutress RI, Beers SA. Obesity is associated with Immunometabolic changes in adipose tissue that may drive treatment resistance in breast cancer: Immune-metabolic reprogramming and novel therapeutic strategies. Cancers. 2023;**15**(9):2440-2440

[42] Hotamisligil GS. Endoplasmic reticulum stress and the inflammatory basis of metabolic disease. Cell. 2010;**140**(6):900-917

[43] Chen IC, Awasthi D, Hsu CL, Song M, Chae CS, Dannenberg AJ, et al. High-fat diet-induced obesity alters dendritic cell homeostasis by enhancing mitochondrial fatty acid oxidation. Journal of Immunology. 2022;**209**(1):69-76

[44] Fujisaka S, Usui I, Ikutani M, Aminuddin A, Takikawa A, Tsuneyama K, et al. Adipose tissue hypoxia induces inflammatory M1 polarity of macrophages in an HIF-1α-dependent and HIF-1α-independent manner in obese mice. Diabetologia. 2013;**56**(6):1403-1412

[45] Chan PC, Lu CH, Chien HC, Tian YF, Hsieh PS. Adipose tissue-derived CCL5 enhances local pro-inflammatory Monocytic MDSCs accumulation and inflammation via CCR5 receptor in high-fat diet-fed mice. International Journal of Molecular Sciences. 2022;**23**(22):14226

[46] Baturcam E, Abubaker J, Tiss A, Abu-Farha M, Khadir A, Al-Ghimlas F, et al. Physical exercise reduces the expression of RANTES and its CCR5 receptor in the adipose tissue of obese humans. Mediators of Inflammation. 2014;**2014**:27150. Available from: https://onlinelibrary.wiley.com/doi/epdf/10.1155/2014/627150

[47] Zhou H, Liao X, Zeng Q, Zhang H, Song J, Hu W, et al. Metabolic effects of CCL5 deficiency in lean and obese mice. Frontiers in Immunology. 2023;**13**:1059687-1059687

[48] Lumeng CN, Bodzin JL, Saltiel AR. Obesity induces a phenotypic switch in adipose tissue macrophage polarization. The Journal of Clinical Investigation. 2007;**117**(1):175-184

[49] Jiao P, Ma J, Feng B, Zhang H, Alan Diehl J, Eugene Chin Y, et al. FFA-induced adipocyte inflammation and insulin resistance: Involvement of ER stress and IKKβ pathways. Obesity. 2011;**19**(3):483-491

[50] Cinti S, Mitchell G, Barbatelli G, Murano I, Ceresi E, Faloia E, et al. Adipocyte death defines macrophage localization and function in adipose tissue of obese mice and humans. Journal of Lipid Research. 2005;**46**(11):2347-2355

[51] Rausch ME, Weisberg S, Vardhana P, Tortoriello DV. Obesity in C57BL/6J mice is characterized by adipose tissue hypoxia and cytotoxic T-cell infiltration. International Journal of Obesity. 2008;**32**(3):451-463

[52] Yin J, Gao Z, He Q, Zhou D, Guo Z, Ye J. Role of hypoxia in obesity-induced disorders of glucose and lipid metabolism in adipose tissue. American Journal of Physiology - Endocrinology and Metabolism. 2009;**296**(2):E333-E342

[53] Milanski M, Degasperi G, Coope A, Morari J, Denis R, Cintra DE, et al. Saturated fatty acids produce an inflammatory response predominantly through the activation of TLR4 signaling in hypothalamus: Implications for the pathogenesis of obesity. The Journal of Neuroscience. 2009;**29**(2):359-370

[54] Strissel KJ, Stancheva Z, Miyoshi H, Perfield JW, DeFuria J, Jick Z, et al. Adipocyte death, adipose tissue remodeling, and obesity complications. Diabetes. 2007;**56**(12):2910-2918

[55] Deshmane SL, Kremlev S, Amini S, Sawaya BE. Monocyte chemoattractant Protein-1 (MCP-1): An overview. Journal of Interferon & Cytokine Research. 2009;**29**(6):313-326

[56] Milner JJ, Beck MA. Micronutrients, immunology and inflammation the impact of obesity on the immune response to infection. The Proceedings of the Nutrition Society. 2012;**71**(2):298-306

[57] Carolan E, Tobin LM, Mangan BA, Corrigan M, Gaoatswe G, Byrne G, et al. Altered distribution and increased IL-17 production by mucosal-associated invariant T cells in adult and childhood obesity. The Journal of Immunology. 2015;**194**(12):5775-5780

[58] Wen H, Gris D, Lei Y, Jha S, Zhang L, Huang MTH, et al. Fatty acid-induced NLRP3-ASC inflammasome activation interferes with insulin signaling. Nature Immunology. 2011;**12**(5):408-415

[59] Silva HM, Báfica A, Rodrigues-Luiz GF, Chi J, Santos d'Emery PA, Reis BS, et al. Vasculature-associated fat macrophages readily adapt to inflammatory and metabolic challenges. Journal of Experimental Medicine. 2019;**216**(4):786-806

[60] Weisberg SP, McCann D, Desai M, Rosenbaum M, Leibel RL, Ferrante AW. Obesity is associated with macrophage accumulation in adipose tissue. The Journal of Clinical Investigation. 2003;**112**(12):1796-1808

[61] Xu H, Barnes GT, Yang Q, Tan G, Yang D, Chou CJ, et al. Chronic inflammation in fat plays a crucial role in the development of obesity-related insulin resistance. The Journal of Clinical Investigation. 2003;**112**(12):1821-1830

[62] Wu Y, Wu C, Shi T, Cai Q, Wang T, Xiong Y, et al. FAP expression in adipose tissue macrophages promotes obesity and metabolic inflammation. National Academy of Sciences of the United States of America. 2023;**120**(51):e2303075120

[63] Brandstadter JD, Yang Y. Natural killer cell responses to viral infection. Journal of Innate Immunity. 2011;**3**(3):274-279

[64] Lynch LA, O'Connell JM, Kwasnik AK, Cawood TJ, O'Farrelly C, O'Shea DB. Are natural killer cells protecting the metabolically healthy obese patient? Obesity. 2009;**17**(3):601-605

[65] Tobin LM, Mavinkurve M, Carolan E, Kinlen D, O'Brien EC, Little MA, et al. NK cells in childhood obesity are activated, metabolically stressed, and functionally deficient. JCI Insight. 2017;**2**(24):e94939

[66] O'Shea D, Hogan AE. Dysregulation of natural killer cells in obesity. Cancers (Basel). 2019;**11**(4):573

[67] Smith AG, Sheridan PA, Harp JB, Beck MA. Diet-induced obese mice have increased mortality and altered immune responses when infected with influenza virus. The Journal of Nutrition. 2007;**137**(5):1236-1243

[68] Liu SY, Sanchez DJ, Aliyari R, Lu S, Cheng G. Systematic identification of type I and type II interferon-induced antiviral factors. Proceedings of the National Academy of Sciences of the United States of America. 2012;**109**(11):4239-4244

[69] Bergin R, Kinlen D, Kedia-Mehta N, Hayes E, Cassidy FC, Cody D, et al. Mucosal-associated invariant T cells are associated with insulin resistance in childhood obesity, and disrupt insulin signalling via IL-17. Diabetologia. 2022;**65**(6):1012-1017

[70] Cassidy FC, Kedia-Mehta N, Bergin R, Woodcock A, Berisha A, Bradley B, et al. Glycogen-fuelled metabolism supports rapid mucosal-associated invariant T cell responses. National Academy of Sciences of the United States of America. 2023;**120**(25):e2300566120

[71] Winer S, Paltser G, Chan Y, Tsui H, Engleman E, Winer D, et al. Obesity predisposes to Th17 bias. European Journal of Immunology. 2009;**39**(9):2629-2635

[72] Sumarac-Dumanovic M, Stevanovic D, Ljubic A, Jorga J, Simic M, Stamenkovic-Pejkovic D, et al. Increased activity of interleukin-23/interleukin-17 proinflammatory axis in obese women. International Journal of Obesity. 2009;**33**(1):151-156

[73] O'Brien A, Loftus RM, Pisarska MM, Tobin LM, Bergin R, Wood NAW, et al. Obesity reduces mTORC1 activity in mucosal-associated invariant T

cells, driving defective metabolic and functional responses. The Journal of Immunology. 2019;**202**(12):3404-3411

[74] Kedia-Mehta N, Pisarska MM, Rollings C, O'Neill C, De Barra C, Foley C, et al. The proliferation of human mucosal-associated invariant T cells requires a MYC-SLC7A5-glycolysis metabolic axis. Science Signaling. 2023;**16**(781). Available from: https://www.science.org/doi/epdf/10.1126/scisignal.abo2709

[75] Rodríguez-Rodríguez E, Salas-González MD, Ortega RM, López-Sobaler AM. Leukocytes and neutrophil–lymphocyte ratio as indicators of insulin resistance in overweight/obese school-children. Frontiers in Nutrition. 2022;**8**:811081

[76] Dixon JB, O'Brien PE. Obesity and the white blood cell count: Changes with sustained weight loss. Obesity Surgery. 2006;**16**(3):251-257

[77] Elgazar-Carmon V, Rudich A, Hadad N, Levy R. Neutrophils transiently infiltrate intra-abdominal fat early in the course of high-fat feeding. Journal of Lipid Research. 2008;**49**(9):1894-1903

[78] McDowell SAC, Luo RBE, Arabzadeh A, Doré S, Bennett NC, Breton V, et al. Neutrophil oxidative stress mediates obesity-associated vascular dysfunction and metastatic transmigration. Nature Cancer. 2021;**2**(5):545-562

[79] Nijhuis J, Rensen SS, Slaats Y, van Dielen FMH, Buurman WA, Greve JWM. Neutrophil activation in morbid obesity, chronic activation of acute inflammation. Obesity. 2009;**17**(11):2014-2018

[80] Banchereau J, Briere F, Caux C, Davoust J, Lebecque S, Liu YJ, et al. Immunobiology of dendritic cells. Annual Review of Immunology. 2000;**18**:767-811

[81] Steinman RM. The dendritic cell system and its role in immunogenicity. Annual Review of Immunology. 1991;**9**(1):271-296

[82] Albert ML, Pearce SFA, Francisco LM, Sauter B, Roy P, Silverstein RL, et al. Immature dendritic cells phagocytose apoptotic cells via $\alpha v\beta 5$ and CD36, and cross-present antigens to cytotoxic T lymphocytes. The Journal of Experimental Medicine. 1998;**188**(7):1359-1368

[83] Ackerman AL, Cresswell P. Regulation of MHC class I transport in human dendritic cells and the dendritic-like cell line KG-1. The Journal of Immunology. 2003;**170**(8):4178-4188

[84] Kim MK, Kim J. Properties of immature and mature dendritic cells: Phenotype, morphology, phagocytosis, and migration. RSC Advances. 2019;**9**(20):11230-11238

[85] Nagorsen D, Marincola FM, Panelli MC. Cytokine and chemokine expression profiles of maturing dendritic cells using multiprotein platform arrays. Cytokine. 2004;**25**(1):31-35

[86] Sallusto F, Lanzavecchia A. The instructive role of dendritic cells on T-cell responses. Arthritis Research & Therapy. 2002;**4**(3):1-6

[87] HJP VDZ, Brombacher EC, Lambooij JM, Pelgrom LR, Zawistowska-Deniziak A, Patente TA, et al. Dendritic cell-intrinsic LKB1-AMPK/SIK signaling controls metabolic homeostasis by limiting the hepatic Th17 response during obesity. JCI Insight. 2023;**8**(11):e157948

[88] Bertola A, Ciucci T, Rousseau D, Bourlier V, Duffaut C, Bonnafous S, et al.

Identification of adipose tissue dendritic cells correlated with obesity-associated insulin-resistance and inducing Th17 responses in mice and patients. Diabetes. 2012;**61**(9):2238-2247

[89] O'Shea D, Corrigan M, Dunne MR, Jackson R, Woods C, Gaoatswe G, et al. Changes in human dendritic cell number and function in severe obesity may contribute to increased susceptibility to viral infection. International Journal of Obesity. 2013;**37**(11):1510-1513

[90] Macdougall CE, Wood EG, Loschko J, Scagliotti V, Cassidy FC, Robinson ME, et al. Visceral adipose tissue immune homeostasis is regulated by the crosstalk between adipocytes and dendritic cell subsets. Cell Metabolism. 2018;**27**(3):588-601

[91] Curtsinger JM, Mescher MF. Inflammatory cytokines as a third signal for T cell activation. Current Opinion in Immunology. 2010;**22**(3):333-340

[92] Medzhitov R, Janeway CA. Innate immunity: Impact on the adaptive immune response. Current Opinion in Immunology. 1997;**9**(1):4-9

[93] Jaiswal AK, Makhija S, Stahr N, Sandey M, Suryawanshi A, Saxena A, et al. Dendritic cell-restricted progenitors contribute to obesity-associated airway inflammation via Adam17-p38 MAPK-dependent pathway. Frontiers in Immunology. 2020;**11**:363

[94] Sheridan PA, Paich HA, Handy J, Karlsson EA, Hudgens MG, Sammon AB, et al. Obesity is associated with impaired immune response to influenza vaccination in humans. International Journal of Obesity. 2012;**36**(8):1072-1077

[95] Smith AG, Sheridan PA, Tseng RJ, Sheridan JF, Beck MA. Selective impairment in dendritic cell function and altered antigen-specific CD8+ T-cell responses in diet-induced obese mice infected with influenza virus. Immunology. 2009;**126**(2):268-279

[96] Cho KW, Zamarron BF, Muir LA, Singer K, Porsche CE, DelProposto JB, et al. Adipose tissue dendritic cells are independent contributors to obesity-induced inflammation and insulin resistance. Journal of Immunology. 2016;**197**(9):3650-3661

[97] Boi SK, Buchta CM, Pearson NA, Francis MB, Meyerholz DK, Grobe JL, et al. Obesity alters immune and metabolic profiles: New insight from obese-resistant mice on high fat diet. Obesity. 2016;**24**(10):2140-2149

[98] Macia L, Delacre M, Abboud G, Ouk TS, Delanoye A, Verwaerde C, et al. Impairment of dendritic cell functionality and steady-state number in obese mice. The Journal of Immunology. 2006;**177**(9):5997-6006

[99] James BR, Tomanek-Chalkley A, Askeland EJ, Kucaba T, Griffith TS, Norian LA. Diet-induced obesity alters dendritic cell function in the presence and absence of tumor growth. Journal of Immunology. 2012;**189**(3):1311-1321

[100] Nishimura S, Manabe I, Nagasaki M, Eto K, Yamashita H, Ohsugi M, et al. CD8+ effector T cells contribute to macrophage recruitment and adipose tissue inflammation in obesity. Nature Medicine. 2009;**15**(8):914-920

[101] Karlsson EA, Sheridan PA, Beck MA. Diet-induced obesity impairs the T cell memory response to influenza virus infection. The Journal of Immunology. 2010;**184**(6):3127-3133

[102] Endo Y, Asou HK, Matsugae N, Hirahara K, Shinoda K, Tumes DJ,

et al. Obesity drives Th17 cell differentiation by inducing the lipid metabolic kinase, ACC1. Cell Reports. 2015;**12**(6):1042-1055

[103] Surendar J, Frohberger SJ, Karunakaran I, Schmitt V, Stamminger W, Neumann AL, et al. Adiponectin limits IFN-γ and IL-17 producing CD4 T cells in obesity by restraining cell intrinsic glycolysis. Frontiers in Immunology. 2019;**10**:2555

[104] Teijaro JR, Verhoeven D, Page CA, Turner D, Farber DL. Memory CD4 T cells direct protective responses to influenza virus in the lungs through helper-independent mechanisms. Journal of Virology. 2010;**84**(18):9217-9226

[105] Russell JH, Ley TJ. Lymphocyte-mediated cytotoxicity. Annual Review of Immunology. 2002;**20**:323-370

[106] Rebeles J, Green WD, Alwarawrah Y, Nichols AG, Eisner W, Danzaki K, et al. Obesity-induced changes in T-cell metabolism are associated with impaired memory T-cell response to influenza and are not reversed with weight loss. The Journal of Infectious Diseases. 2019;**219**(10):1652-1661

[107] Norell H, Da Palma TM, Lesher A, Kaur N, Mehrotra M, Naga OS, et al. Inhibition of superoxide generation upon TCR engagement rescues Mart-127-35 reactive T cells from activation induced cell death. Cancer Research. 2009;**69**(15):6282-6289

[108] Case AJ, McGill JL, Tygrett LT, Shirasawa T, Spitz DR, Waldschmidt TJ, et al. Elevated mitochondrial superoxide disrupts normal T-cell development, impairing adaptive immune responses to an influenza challenge. Free Radical Biology and Medicine. 2011;**50**(3):448-458

[109] Weatherill AR, Lee JY, Zhao L, Lemay DG, Youn HS, Hwang DH. Saturated and polyunsaturated fatty acids reciprocally modulate dendritic cell functions mediated through TLR4. The Journal of Immunology. 2005;**174**(9):5390-5397

[110] Nieto-Vazquez I, Fernández-Veledo S, Krämer DK, Vila-Bedmar R, Garcia-Guerra L, Lorenzo M. Insulin resistance associated to obesity: The link TNF-alpha. Archives of Physiology and Biochemistry. 2008;**114**(3):183-194

[111] Laplante M, Sabatini DM. mTOR signaling at a glance. Journal of Cell Science. 2009;**122**(20):3589-3594

[112] Shaw RJ. LKB1 and AMPK control of mTOR signalling and growth. Acta Physiologica. 2009;**196**(1):65-80

[113] Deiuliis J, Shah Z, Shah N, Needleman B, Mikami D, Narula V, et al. Visceral adipose inflammation in obesity is associated with critical alterations in Tregulatory cell numbers. PLoS One. 2011;**6**(1):e16376

[114] Feuerer M, Shen Y, Littman DR, Benoist C, Mathis D. How punctual ablation of regulatory T cells unleashes an autoimmune lesion within the pancreatic islets. Immunity. 2009;**31**(4):654-664

[115] Wagner NM, Brandhorst G, Czepluch F, Lankeit M, Eberle C, Herzberg S, et al. Circulating regulatory T cells are reduced in obesity and may identify subjects at increased metabolic and cardiovascular risk. Obesity. 2013;**21**(3):461-468

[116] Costanzo AE, Taylor KR, Dutt S, Han PP, Fujioka K, Jameson JM. Obesity impairs γδ T cell homeostasis and antiviral function in humans. PLoS One. 2015;**10**(3):e0120918

[117] Wijngaarden LH, van der Harst E, Klaassen RA, Dunkelgrun M, Kuijper TM, Klepper M, et al. Effects of morbid obesity and metabolic syndrome on the composition of circulating immune subsets. Frontiers in Immunology. 2021;**12**:675018

[118] Wijngaarden LH, Taselaar AE, Nuijten F, Van Der Harst E, Klaassen RA, Kuijper TM, et al. T and B cell composition and cytokine producing capacity before and after bariatric surgery. Frontiers in Immunology. 2022;**13**:888278

[119] Šlisere B, Arisova M, Aizbalte O, Salmiņa MM, Zolovs M, Levenšteins M, et al. Distinct B cell profiles characterise healthy weight and obesity pre- and post-bariatric surgery. International Journal of Obesity. 2023;**47**(10):970-978

[120] Harris A. Hepatitis B. CDC Yellow Book 2024 [Internet]. Available from: https://wwwnc.cdc.gov/travel/yellowbook/2024/infections-diseases/hepatitis-b [Accessed: February 13, 2025].

[121] Ikuta KS, Swetschinski LR, Aguilar GR, Sharara F, Mestrovic T, Gray AP, et al. Global mortality associated with 33 bacterial pathogens in 2019: A systematic analysis for the global burden of disease study 2019. The Lancet. 2022;**400**(10369):2221-2248

[122] Poostchi M, Silamut K, Maude RJ, Jaeger S, Thoma G. Image analysis and machine learning for detecting malaria. Translational Research. 2018;**194**:36-55

[123] Hemelaar J, Elangovan R, Yun J, Dickson-Tetteh L, Fleminger I, Kirtley S, et al. Global and regional molecular epidemiology of HIV-1, 1990-2015: A systematic review, global survey, and trend analysis. The Lancet Infectious Diseases. 2019;**19**(2):143-155

[124] Mathers C, Stevens G, Hogan D, Mahanani WR, Ho J. Global and regional causes of death: Patterns and trends, 2000-15. In: Jamison DT, Gelband H, Horton S, Jha P, Laxminarayan R, Mock CN, et al., editors. Disease Control Priorities: Improving Health and Reducing Poverty. 3rd ed. Washington (DC): The International Bank for Reconstruction and Development/The World Bank; 2017

[125] Naghavi M, Mestrovic T, Gray A, Hayoon AG, Swetschinski LR, Aguilar GR, et al. Global burden associated with 85 pathogens in 2019: A systematic analysis for the global burden of disease study 2019. The Lancet Infectious Diseases. 2024;**24**(8):868-895

[126] Romanello M, Napoli CD, Drummond P, Green C, Kennard H, Lampard P, et al. The 2022 report of the lancet countdown on health and climate change: Health at the mercy of fossil fuels. The Lancet. 2022;**400**(10363):1619-1654

[127] Oliveira M, Antunes W, Mota S, Madureira-Carvalho Á, Dinis-Oliveira RJ, Dias da Silva D. An overview of the recent advances in antimicrobial resistance. Microorganisms. 2024;**12**(9):1920

[128] Jiang J, Qin X, Liu H, Meng S, Abdullah AS, Huang J, et al. An optimal BMI range associated with a lower risk of mortality among HIV-infected adults initiating antiretroviral therapy in Guangxi, China. Scientific Reports. 2019;**9**(1):7816

[129] Sharma A, Hoover DR, Shi Q, Gustafson D, Plankey MW, Hershow RC, et al. Relationship between body mass index and mortality in HIV-infected HAART users in the Women's interagency HIV study. PLoS One. 2015;**10**(12):e0143740

[130] Yu MW, Shih WL, Lin CL, Liu CJ, Jian JW, Tsai KS, et al. Body-mass index and progression of hepatitis B: A population-based cohort study in men. Journal of Clinical Oncology. 2008;**26**(34):5576-5582

[131] Nickbakhsh S, Leitch ECM, Smith S, Davis C, Hutchinson S, Irving WL, et al. Geographical variation in hepatitis C-related severe liver disease and patient risk factors: A multicentre cross-sectional study. Epidemiology & Infection. 2023;**151**:e59

[132] Divella R, Mazzocca A, Daniele A, Sabbà C, Paradiso A. Obesity, nonalcoholic fatty liver disease and Adipocytokines network in promotion of cancer. International Journal of Biological Sciences. 2019;**15**(3):610-616

[133] Ye Q, Zou B, Yeo YH, Li J, Huang DQ, Wu Y, et al. Global prevalence, incidence, and outcomes of non-obese or lean non-alcoholic fatty liver disease: A systematic review and meta-analysis. The Lancet Gastroenterology & Hepatology. 2020;**5**(8):739-752

[134] Maccioni L, Weber S, Elgizouli M, Stoehlker AS, Geist I, Peter HH, et al. Obesity and risk of respiratory tract infections: Results of an infection-diary based cohort study. BMC Public Health. 2018;**18**:1-13

[135] Jedrychowski W, Maugeri U, Flak E, Mroz E, Bianchi I. Predisposition to acute respiratory infections among overweight preadolescent children: An epidemiologic study in Poland. Public Health. 1998;**112**(3):189-195

[136] Fiore AE, Uyeki TM, Broder K, Finelli L, Euler GL, Singleton JA, et al. Prevention and control of influenza with vaccines: Recommendations of the advisory committee on immunization practices (ACIP). MMWR - Recommendations and Reports. 2010;**59**(RR-8):1-62

[137] Fezeu L, Julia C, Henegar A, Bitu J, Hu FB, Grobbee DE, et al. Obesity is associated with higher risk of intensive care unit admission and death in influenza a (H1N1) patients: A systematic review and meta-analysis. Obesity Reviews. 2011;**12**(8):653-659

[138] Simonnet A, Chetboun M, Poissy J, Raverdy V, Noulette J, Duhamel A, et al. High prevalence of obesity in severe acute respiratory syndrome Coronavirus-2 (SARS-CoV-2) requiring invasive mechanical ventilation. Obesity. 2020;**28**(7):1195-1199

[139] Choban PS, Heckler R, Burge JC, Flancbaum L. Increased incidence of nosocomial infections in obese surgical patients. The American Surgeon. 1995;**61**(11):1001-1005

[140] Badawi A, Ryoo SG. Prevalence of comorbidities in the Middle East respiratory syndrome coronavirus (MERS-CoV): A systematic review and meta-analysis. International Journal of Infectious Diseases. 2016;**49**:129-133

[141] Wahl TS, Patel FC, Goss LE, Chu DI, Grams J, Morris MS. The obese colorectal surgery patient: Surgical site infection and outcomes. Diseases of the Colon & Rectum. 2018;**61**(8):938-945

[142] Merkow RP, Bilimoria KY, McCarter MD, Bentrem DJ. Effect of body mass index on short-term outcomes after colectomy for cancer. Journal of the American College of Surgeons. 2009;**208**(1):53-61

[143] Paulsen J, Askim Å, Mohus RM, Mehl A, Dewan A, Solligård E, et al. Associations of obesity and lifestyle with the risk and mortality of bloodstream

infection in a general population: A 15-year follow-up of 64 027 individuals in the HUNT study. International Journal of Epidemiology. 2017;**46**(5):1573-1581

[144] Jansåker F, Forsberg PO, Li X, Sundquist K. The relation of body mass index, body height, and parity to pyelonephritis: A nationwide population-based cohort study of over one million parous women (1997-2018). International Journal of Infectious Diseases. 2022;**125**:67-73

[145] Vessey MP, Metcalfe MA, McPherson K, Yeates D. Urinary tract infection in relation to diaphragm use and obesity. International Journal of Epidemiology. 1987;**16**(3):441-444

[146] Nassaji M, Ghorbani R, Tamadon MR, Bitaraf M. Association between body mass index and urinary tract infection in adult patients. Nephro-Urology Monthly. 2015;**7**(1):e22712

[147] Weng L, Fan J, Yu C, Guo Y, Bian Z, Wei Y, et al. Body-mass index and long-term risk of sepsis-related mortality: A population-based cohort study of 0.5 million Chinese adults. Critical Care. 2020;**24**(1):534

[148] Pitts SI, Maruthur NM, Langley GE, Pondo T, Shutt KA, Hollick R, et al. Obesity, diabetes, and the risk of invasive group B streptococcal disease in nonpregnant adults in the United States. Open Forum Infectious Diseases. 2018;**5**(6):ofy030

[149] Frasca D, McElhaney J. Influence of obesity on pneumococcus infection risk in the elderly. Frontiers in Endocrinology. 2019;**10**:71

[150] Langley G, Hao Y, Pondo T, Miller L, Petit S, Thomas A, et al. The impact of obesity and diabetes on the risk of disease and death due to invasive group a streptococcus infections in adults. Clinical Infectious Diseases. 2016;**62**(7):845-852

[151] Olsen K, Danielsen K, Wilsgaard T, Sangvik M, Sollid JUE, Thune I, et al. Obesity and Staphylococcus aureus nasal colonization among women and men in a general population. PLoS One. 2013;**8**(5):e63716

[152] Befus M, Lowy FD, Miko BA, Mukherjee DV, Herzig CTA, Larson EL. Obesity as a determinant of Staphylococcus aureus colonization among inmates in maximum-security prisons in New York state. American Journal of Epidemiology. 2015;**182**(6):494-502

[153] Lönnroth K, Williams BG, Cegielski P, Dye C. A consistent log-linear relationship between tuberculosis incidence and body mass index. International Journal of Epidemiology. 2010;**39**(1):149-155

[154] Yen YF, Hu HY, Lee YL, Ku PW, Lin IF, Chu D, et al. Obesity/overweight reduces the risk of active tuberculosis: A nationwide population-based cohort study in Taiwan. International Journal of Obesity. 2017;**41**(6):971-975

[155] Cho SH, Lee H, Kwon H, Shin DW, Joh HK, Han K, et al. Association of underweight status with the risk of tuberculosis: A nationwide population-based cohort study. Scientific Reports. 2022;**12**(1):16207

[156] Choi H, Yoo JE, Han K, Choi W, Rhee SY, Lee H, et al. Body mass index, diabetes, and risk of tuberculosis: A retrospective cohort study. Frontiers in Nutrition. 2021;**8**:739766

[157] Wyss K, Wångdahl A, Vesterlund M, Hammar U, Dashti S, Naucler P, et al. Obesity and diabetes as risk factors for

severe plasmodium falciparum malaria: Results from a Swedish Nationwide study. Clinical Infectious Diseases. 2017;**65**(6):949-958

[158] Brown L, Datta D, Bond C, Namazzi R, Opoka R, John C. Underweight is associated with mortality among Ugandan children with plasmodium falciparum severe malaria. Insight: Indiana University Medical Student Research Journal. 2021;**4**(1):74

[159] Kojom Foko LP, Nolla NP, Nyabeyeu Nyabeyeu H, Tonga C, Lehman LG. Prevalence, patterns, and determinants of malaria and malnutrition in Douala, Cameroon: A cross-sectional community-based study. BioMed Research International. 2021;**1**:5553344

[160] Clem AS. Fundamentals of vaccine immunology. Journal of Global Infectious Diseases. 2011;**3**(1):73-78

[161] Thomas PG, Keating R, Hulse-Post DJ, Doherty PC. Cell-mediated protection in influenza infection. Emerging Infectious Diseases. 2006;**12**(1):48-54

[162] Carrat F, Flahault A. Influenza vaccine: The challenge of antigenic drift. Vaccine. 2007;**25**(39-40):6852-6862

[163] Karlsson EA, Sheridan PA, Beck MA. Diet-induced obesity in mice reduces the maintenance of influenza-specific CD8+ memory T cells. The Journal of Nutrition. 2010;**140**(9):1691-1697

[164] Berger S, Polotsky VY. Leptin and leptin resistance in the pathogenesis of obstructive sleep apnea: A possible link to oxidative stress and cardiovascular complications. Oxidative Medicine and Cellular Longevity. 2018;**2018**(1):5137947

[165] Pérez-Pérez A, Vilariño-García T, Fernández-Riejos P, Martín-González J, Segura-Egea JJ, Sánchez-Margalet V. Role of leptin as a link between metabolism and the immune system. Cytokine & Growth Factor Reviews. 2017;**35**:71-84

[166] Mackey-Lawrence NM, Petri WA. Leptin and mucosal immunity. Mucosal Immunology. 2012;**5**(5):472-479

[167] Stonier SW, Ma LJ, Castillo EF, Schluns KS. Dendritic cells drive memory CD8 T-cell homeostasis via IL-15 transpresentation. Blood. 2008;**112**(12):4546-4554

[168] Lawrence VJ, Kopelman PG. Medical consequences of obesity. Clinics in Dermatology. 2004;**22**(4):296-302

[169] Kwon Y, Jeong SJ. Association between body mass index and hepatitis B antibody seropositivity in children. Korean Journal of Pediatrics. 2019;**62**(11):416-421

[170] Eliakim A, Swindt C, Zaldivar F, Casali P, Cooper DM. Reduced tetanus antibody titers in overweight children. Autoimmunity. 2006;**39**(2):137-141

[171] Onyango TB, Zhou F, Bredholt G, Brokstad KA, Lartey S, Mohn KGI, et al. SARS-CoV-2 specific immune responses in overweight and obese COVID-19 patients. Frontiers in Immunology. 2023;**14**:1287388

[172] Wrigley Kelly NE, Kenny G, Cassidy FC, Garcia-Leon AA, De Barra C, Mallon PWG, et al. Individuals with obesity who survive SARS-CoV-2 infection have preserved antigen-specific T cell frequencies. Obesity. 2022;**30**(10):1927-1931

[173] Vimercati L, De Maria L, Quarato M, Caputi A, Gesualdo L, Migliore G, et al. Association between long COVID and overweight/

obesity. Journal of Clinical Medicine. 2021;**10**(18):4143

[174] Ou X, Jiang J, Lin B, Liu Q, Lin W, Chen G, et al. Antibody responses to COVID-19 vaccination in people with obesity: A systematic review and meta-analysis. Influenza and Other Respiratory Viruses. 2023;**17**(1):e13078

[175] Wrigley Kelly NE, De Barra C, Shaamile F, Holland A, Shaw L, Mallon PWG, et al. Antigen specific T cells in people with obesity at five months following ChAdOx1 COVID-19 vaccination. International Journal of Obesity. 2023;**47**(1):83-86

[176] Neidich SD, Green WD, Rebeles J, Karlsson EA, Schultz-Cherry S, Noah TL, et al. Increased risk of influenza among vaccinated adults who are obese. International Journal of Obesity. 2017;**41**(9):1324-1330

[177] Sbraccia P, Dicker D. Obesity is a chronic progressive relapsing disease of particular interest for internal medicine. Internal and Emergency Medicine. 2023;**18**(1):1-5

[178] Kolotkin RL, Andersen JR. A systematic review of reviews: Exploring the relationship between obesity, weight loss and health-related quality of life. Clinical Obesity. 2017;**7**(5):273-289

[179] Peeters A, Barendregt JJ, Willekens F, Mackenbach JP, Al Mamun A, Bonneux L, et al. Obesity in adulthood and its consequences for life expectancy: A life-table analysis. Annals of Internal Medicine. 2003;**138**(1):24-32

[180] Maier HE, Lopez R, Sanchez N, Ng S, Gresh L, Ojeda S, et al. Obesity increases the duration of influenza a virus shedding in adults. The Journal of Infectious Diseases. 2018;**218**(9):1378-1382

Chapter 4

Lipedema Adipocytes in Culture: Signs of Hypertrophy, Inflammation, and Fibrosis

Anna Maria Ernst, Erwin Schimak, Marianne Steiner, Anna-Theresa Lipp, Hans-Christian Bauer and Hannelore Bauer

Abstract

Despite extensive research during the last couple of years, lipedema still appears enigmatic in respect to its pathogenesis. In our in vitro study, we have set out to further characterize lipedema adipocytes, concentrating on gene and protein expression, which might help to develop ideas explaining the excessive accumulation of adipose tissue in women with lipedema. Using 2D cultures we show that gene expression in lipedema and non-lipedema adipocytes differs significantly in terms of genes related to lipid droplet size determination, insulin signaling and glucose uptake. A pronounced hypertrophy, recognizable by a significantly increased average lipid droplet size, was visible in differentiated lipedema adipocytes grown in 3D cultures. In addition, gene and protein expression related to inflammation and fibrosis were upregulated in lipedema adipocytes compared to controls, supporting earlier reports. Taken together, results from our in vitro studies suggest that lipedema adipose cells are capable of retaining their hypertrophic nature under culture conditions and open new aspects focusing on insulin signaling and PDGFRA-mediated balancing of adipogenic versus fibrogenic differentiation of lipedema adipose tissue.

Keywords: lipedema, adipose tissue-derived stromal cells, gene expression, adipogenic differentiation, inflammation, hypertrophy, lipid droplet size

1. Introduction

According to the current state of knowledge, lipedema can be classified as a fat distribution disorder—a term usually describing the localized imbalance of subcutaneous fat deposition and affecting both overweight and normal-weight individuals.

Women who suffer from lipedema (synonymously also referred to as adiposis dolorosa or lipalgia) experience a symmetrical enlargement of their extremities, with partial involvement of the hips and buttocks at advanced stages, while their waists remain disproportionately small [1–6]. Lipedema can occur as both a syndromic and non-syndromic disease, with a suggested but yet-undefined autosomal dominant inheritance [7, 8].

Apart from the unbalanced accumulation of subcutaneous fat on the extremities, people with lipedema show several pathological characteristics such as tenderness, pressure pain, easy bruising and depressive moods, while suffering from an inexorable, diet- and exercise-resistant weight gain [9].

Lipedema is not typically associated with metabolic complications and related cardiovascular diseases, while hypothyroidism appears to be a frequent co-morbidity of lipedema [10], particularly at higher stages.

Lipedema is found predominantly, if not exclusively, in women, the onset being associated with major hormonal changes. In this context, puberty seems to be a significant trigger for lipedema, followed by pregnancy and menopause, apart from other, less defined, causes.

The rare occurrence of lipedema in men is usually a consequence of a primary hormonal disorder [7]. However, despite the many indications that lipedema might be an estrogen-associated disease [11], scientific evidence clearly demonstrating a causal role for estrogen in the initiation or progression of lipedema is still missing.

One important key detail distinguishing lipedema from other fat distribution disorders such as Madelung's disease (multiple symmetric lipomatosis), Dercum's disease, or familial multiple lipomatosis, is the higher relative frequency with which it occurs [12]. While the above-mentioned diseases are particularly rare, the prevalence of lipedema is estimated up to 11% in women and post-pubertal girls [13]. However, statistic numbers concerning the prevalence of lipedema vary substantially [14]. This can be explained by the limited availability of accurate diagnostic options, the lack of molecular "markers" and probably by a long-standing ignorance of this disease. In addition, lipedema has often been misdiagnosed as obesity, lymphatic or venous insufficiency, or lipohypertrophy, which is not surprising given the phenotypic similarities and the partially shared symptomatology at advanced stages [15–17].

It needs to be emphasized that lipohypertrophy differs from lipedema in several important aspects, above all the absence of pain and the weaker (or even absent) tendency to develop edema at advanced stages. Histological and molecular characteristics to distinguish lipohypertrophy from lipedema and secondary lymphedema were recently described [18].

Since lipedema was originally described as a "syndrome characterized by fat legs and orthostatic edema" [19], the assumption that lipedema is triggered by the formation of edema was obvious. Since then, numerous studies have focused on the potential occurrence of lymphatic disturbances and vascular fragility in people with lipedema, with contradicting results (reviewed in [20–22]).

Taking together all evidence available so far, it may be postulated that edema is not integral to the initiation and early development of lipedema. However, during advanced stages, the co-occurrence of obesity and lymphatic impediment is frequently observed. Therefore, conservative treatment including decongestion therapy often achieves success in relieving the patient's pain, but does not impact the pathogenesis of lipedema itself. Currently, liposuction appears to be the best treatment for long-term improvement [23].

The criteria used for the diagnosis of lipedema were established in the 1950s [19] and, with a few modifications introduced by Herbst [24], are still valid today. A thorough visual inspection, palpation and a detailed discussion of the patients' histories are still the basis of daily routine diagnosis. Sonography may improve diagnosis and help to distinguish lipedema from lymphedema, particularly at advanced stages [25].

Although it is generally agreed upon that lipedema progresses through stages [26] that can develop with different dynamics, the biological mechanism(s) underlying this progression are not yet clear. Numerous studies were conducted to explore potential molecular alterations distinguishing lipedema from non-lipedema adipose tissue in vivo and in vitro (reviewed in [21, 22]). Thereby, a major focus was set on the appearance of hyperplasia and hypertrophy, two basic mechanisms underlying adipose tissue accumulation [27, 28], and on the role of low-level inflammation and fibrotic changes in the development of lipedema [29].

Concerning adipose tissue hyperplasia, in vitro studies have contradicted each other. Several articles state that lipedema preadipocytes show increased proliferative activity compared to non-lipedema cells, estimated either upon expression of gene markers such as CD90 or cyclin D1, or using cell counting and metabolic activity assays, while other studies do not support this notion [30–34].

Data concerning the occurrence of hypertrophy in lipedema adipose tissue are more consistent, as demonstrated by the measurements of adipocyte size in biopsied subcutaneous adipose tissue [18, 30, 35, 36]. While it appears plausible that adipocyte size is increased in lipedema adipose tissue, a more detailed analysis supporting this finding is missing. Since most of the molecular data available so far have emerged from studies using in vitro differentiated adipocytes grown from the stromal vascular fraction (SVF) of subcutaneous adipose tissue, it should be clarified, whether the suggested hypertrophy found in vivo is also evident in vitro.

The goal of this study was to further elucidate the previously suggested hypertrophy of lipedema adipocytes using 2D and 3D culture systems. Here we show for the first time that lipedema adipose cells are capable of retaining their hypertrophic nature during cultivation, which is reflected by significantly increased average size of lipid droplets (LDs) in lipedema adipocytes compared to controls. This is supported by our results from gene expression studies showing elevated expression of genes related to LD enlargement in lipedema adipocytes in vitro. In addition, we confirmed the significant upregulation of fibrosis and inflammation-related gene and protein expression in lipedema adipocytes, supporting the notion that lipedema pathology is obviously accompanied and intensified by low-level inflammation and fibrotic alterations.

2. Material and methods

2.1 Human tissue specimens

In vitro experiments were performed on adipose tissue-derived stromal cells (ASCs) isolated from lipoaspirates obtained exclusively from the thigh region of anonymized female donors during routine operations. Ex vivo experiments were performed on tissue excised from cannula incision sites directly before the operations.

Informed consent was acquired from all patients. All experimental protocols concerning human adipose tissues (biopsied material and lipoaspirate) were approved by the Ethics Committee of Salzburg, Austria.

The anonymized donors were categorized into lipedema and control donors: Obese (in the following referred to as OB) lipedema donors (n = 5, average age at operation 29.4 ± 1.5 years, BMI 36.2 ± 4.6 kg/m^2, non-obese (normal weight and overweight, in the following referred to as NW/OW) lipedema donors (n = 10, average age at operation 31.0 ± 6.9 years, BMI 24.4 ± 2.3 kg/m^2), and controls (n = 6, average age at operation 33.4 ± 8.4 years, BMI (25.4 ± 2.1 kg/m^2).

2.2 Cell isolation

SVF from lipoaspirates was isolated according to a standardized procedure. To summarize: To isolate the ASCs, 0.1% collagenase A (Sigma-Aldrich; Vienna, Austria) was dissolved in phosphate buffered saline (PBS). Collagenase solution and lipoaspirate were mixed one to one and incubated for 30 min at 37°C in a water bath under constant agitation. StemMACS MSC expansion medium (MiltenyiBiotech; Bergisch-Gladbach, Germany) was used to stop the collagenase digestion. Supernatant was discarded after centrifugation (340 g) for 10 min, and the pellet was resuspended in PBS and filtered through a 100 μm cell strainer (Falcon; Corning, NY, USA). The pellet was resuspended in culture medium after a second identical centrifugation step before seeding in culture flasks. Whenever necessary, pellets were also washed with red blood cell lysis buffer (RBC lysis buffer, Roche Diagnostics; Rotkreuz, Switzerland), centrifuged again, resuspended in culture medium, and seeded.

After isolation, the ASCs were cultured in basic medium containing high-glucose (4.5 g/L D-Glucose) DMEM with glutamine (Sigma-Aldrich), 10% fetal bovine serum (FBS, Sigma-Aldrich) and 1% antibiotic/antimycotic solution (Sigma-Aldrich). The ASCs were fed once per week and passaged 0–3 times before being used for 2D or 3D experimentation.

2.3 In vitro differentiation

Adipogenic differentiation was induced by switching out basic medium with differentiation and then maintenance medium changes every 3–4 days for 21 days. The differentiation medium ingredients were as follows: DMEM high glucose, 1 μmol/L dexamethasone (Sigma-Aldrich), 0.5 mmol/L 3-isobutyl-1-methylxanthine (IBMX) (Sigma), 10 μg/mL insulin (Sigma-Aldrich) and 100 μmol/L indomethacin (Sigma-Aldrich). The cells were cultured for 4 days in the differentiation medium and then differentiation was maintained for 3 days with DMEM high glucose with the addition of 10 μg/mL insulin, before being cultured with differentiation medium again.

After 21 days, the adipogenic differentiation was verified by Oil Red O (ORO) staining. The cell yield was fixed with 4% paraformaldehyde (PFA), stained with a 60% ORO solution (Sigma-Aldrich), and washed 3× with dH_2O to visualize the red-stained LDs.

2.4 Total RNA extraction and reverse transcription of 2D ASCs

After isolation, seeding in T25 culture flasks, and 21-day adipogenic differentiation induction after confluency, differentiated cells were harvested and homogenized in TRIzol™ Reagent (ThermoFisher Scientific; Waltham, MA, USA). RNA was extracted using the manufacture's protocol. RNA pellets were solubilized in 20–30 μl nuclease-free H_2O (IDT) with 1 μl (1:20 dilution) of RNAase inhibitor (Sigma-Aldrich). RNA yield and quality using the 260/280 nm ratio was established with the NanoDrop 2000c Spectrophotometer (ThermoFisher Scientific).

Reverse transcription was then performed using the iScript™ cDNA synthesis kit (BIORAD; Ipswich, MA, USA) according to the manufacturer's protocol. 1 μg of RNA was used for the cDNA synthesis.

2.5 Quantitative PCR analysis

Quantitative PCRs (qPCRs) were performed with the Luna® Universal Probe qPCR Master Mix (New England Biolabs®; Ipswich, MA, USA) according to the manufacturer's instructions. A concentration of 5 ng/μl cDNA was analyzed per well. Predesigned qPCR assays were selected using Integrated DNA Technologies (IDT; Coralville, IW, USA). **Table 1** lists the primers of the predesigned assays.

All samples were run in technical duplicates and CQ values were analyzed using qBaseplus v2.4 (Biogazelle; Zwijnaarde, Belgium). Relative gene expressions of the data were calculated by normalizing the data to the expression of three reference genes (TBP, PUM1, and RPLP0) which were stably expressed across sample conditions.

2.6 Immunofluorescence staining of cultured cells

SVF-cells were harvested and cultured as described previously. Passage 2 cells were seeded on glass coverslips and grown until confluence. Then, cells were fixed in situ with 4% PFA, and washed with PBS. After permeabilizing with 0.2% TritonX100 and blocking unspecific binding sites by preincubation with 1% Bovine Serum Albumin (BSA) in PBS + 0.05% Tween 20 (PBST) for 30 min, cells were incubated overnight at 4°C with the specific antibodies mo-anti CD68 RTU (#514H12 Bond/Leica; Wetzlar, Germany) mixed with rb-anti CD163 1:75 (#STJ110681, St. Johns; London, UK) diluted in 0.1% PBST. After 4× washing, cells were incubated with the secondary antibody mix of Alexa Fluor® 488 Donkey anti-mouse IgG (H + L) 1:500 and Alexa Fluor® 568 Donkey anti-rabbit IgG (H + L) 1:1500 (both Invitrogen; Waltham, MA, USA) diluted in 0.1% PBST for 30 min at room temperature. Following washing, cell nuclei were stained with DAPI (Sigma-Aldrich) for 10 min.

Cells on coverslips were mounted with CitiFluor™ (Electron Microscopy Sciences; Hatfield, PA, USA) on glass slides. For evaluation of M1 and M2 macrophage-distribution, fluorescence micrographs were taken through a 40× objective with Nikon NIS Elements B software at a Nikon Eclipse 800 microscope equipped with a Nikon DS-Ri1 camera (Nikon; Tokyo, Japan).

Micrographs from 5 to 12 fields (depending on cell density) were taken and nuclei were counted. Overlay pictures of the three channels DAPI, CD68 → green (488 nm) and CD163 → red (568 nm) were assembled with Adobe Photoshop software. CD68 alone and CD68/CD163 positive cells were counted and evaluated in percentages in comparison to DAPI positive cells.

2.7 Spheroid formation, in vitro differentiation and immunofluorescence staining

For morphologic measurements, 6000 ASCs originating from lipedema and control SVF were seeded first in hanging droplets. In short, droplets of 20 μl cell suspension were placed on the underside of a lid of a 30 mm dish, which was then immediately flipped over back on to the dish. The subsequently formed hanging droplets incubated in a 37°C CO_2 incubator for 24 h where aggregation of ASCs was induced. After spheroid formation, the spheroids were transferred to non-adhesive 24-well plates (Nunclon-Sphera; Waltham, MA, USA). Growth of ASC spheroids was monitored throughout 3 days, with daily photographic documentation using a Zeiss Axiovert™ microscope and a GryphaxR Subra camera (Jenoptik; Jena, Germany).

Function	Target gene symbol	Target gene names	ID	Primer 1 sequence; primer 2 sequence; probe
Extracellular matrix organization	COL1A1	Collagen I	NM_000088	5′-CCAGTGTCTCCCTTGGGT-3′; 5′-TGACGAGACCAAGAACTGC-3′; 5′-/56-FAM/ACCCACCGA/Zen/CCAAGAAACCACC /3IABkFQ/-3′
Receptors, growth factors, cofactors, and transporters	GLUT4 (SLC2A4)	Insulin-regulated glucose transporter	NM_001042	5′-TCCTTGCTGTGTTCTCGC-3′; 5′-CCCAGCCACGTCTCATTG-3′; 5′-/56-FAM/TGCCCCZVS/ZEN/GAAGGTGATTGAACAG/3IAVkGQ/-3′
	IGF-1R	Insulin growth like factor 1 receptor	NM_000875	5′-ATCCGCCATTCTCATGCC-3′; 5′-CCAGTCCCACAGTTGCTG-3′; 5′-/56-FAM/ACTCCTTCT/ZEN/ACGTCCTCGACAACCA/3IABkFQ/-3′
	INSR	Insulin receptor	NM_001079817	5′-AAGTGCATCCCTGAGTGTC-3′; 5′-TGGTCTTCTCGCCTTCTAGG-3′; 5′-/56-FAM/TCCCTGTCC/ZEN/CAAGGTGTGCC/3IABkFQ/-3′
	PPARGC1A	Protein alpha PPARG Coactivator 1 Alpha	NM_013261	5′-AGACGTGACCACTGACAATG-3′; 5′-CCACTGCATTCATTATAACTTAGCTG-3′; 5′-/5 g-FAM/CACCCAGG/ZEN/AGGCAGAAGAGC/3IABkGQ/-3′
Components involved in adipogenesis and lipid metabolism	ABHD5 (CGI-58)	Alpha/beta hydrolase domain-containing protein 5	NM_016006	5′-CTGCTTACTCGCTGAAGTACC-3′;5′-TGGATTGGTCTGTCTTGATCAG-3′; 5′/56-FAM/CCCCAAGGC/ZEN/TCCACTAAAATGAGATGA/3IABkFQ/-3′
	AKR1C1	Aldo-Keto Reductase 1C1	NM_001353	5′-TCTATGCTGGTGACTGGACA-3′; 5′-GGCTTTGCTGTAGCTTGC-3′; 5′-56-FAM/CCTCTGGTT/ZEN/AAATCTCTCCTGXTTGGTG/3IABFQ7-3′
	ATGL (PLNPA2)	Adipose triglyceride lipase	NM_020376	5′-CACTGTGATGGTGTTCTTAAGC-3′: 5′-GAGCTCTCATCCAGGCCAAT-3′: 5′-/56-FAM/TGGTGGCAT/Zen/TTCAGACAACCTGC/3IABkFQ/-3′
	CIDEA	Cell Death Inducing DFFA Like Effector A	NR_036468	5′-CAATGACGAATGTTGAAGATGCT-3′; 5′-CCCACTTCATGTACCACCAA-3′; 5′-/56-FAM/ACCCACTCCT/ZEN/GAGCAGCGTGAC/3IABkFQ/-3′
	FSP27 (CIDEC)	Fat-specific protein 27	NM_022094	5′-GACACTCTGATGCTGGCA-3′; GTACTCTTCTGTCTCTACAGTTGTG-3″; 5′-56-FAM/AAGCCCTCTC/ZEN/TTCCTGGTGCTGG/3IABkFQ/-3′
	LPL	Lipoprotein lipase	NM_000237	5′-CTGACTCTGGCCGTGTG-3′; 5′-GGAATGAGGTGGCAAGTGT-3′; 5′-/56-FAM/AGAGTCTGA/ZEN/CCGCCTCCCG/3IABkFQ/-3′
	PLIN1	Perilipin 1	NM_002666	5′-CTGAAGGGCGTTACTGACAA-3′; 5′-CTGGTGGGTTGTCGATGT-3′; 5′-/56-FAM/CCAGGCTGT/ZEN/CGCTGATGGAGC/3IABkFQ/-3′
Cytokine	IL6	Interleukin-6	NM_000600	5′-GCAGATGAGTACAAAGTCCTGA-3′; 5′-TTCTGTGCCTGAGCTTC-3′; 5′-56-FAM/CAACCACAA/ZEN/ATGCCAGCCTGCT/3IABkFQ/-3′

Function	Target gene symbol	Target gene names	ID	Primer 1 sequence; primer 2 sequence; probe
Tissue fibrosis related markers	PDGFRA	Platelet derived growth factor receptor alpha	NM_006206	5′-GCGACAAGGTATAATGGCAGA-3′; 5′-AGACAGAAGAGAATGAGCTTGAAG-3′; 5′-/56-FAM/AGGCTACAT/Zen/CTGGGTCTGGCAC/3IABkFQ/-3′
Reference genes	TBP	TATA-Box binding protein	NM_003194	5′-GATAAGAGAGCCACGAACCAC-3′; 5′-CAAGAACTTAGCTGGAAAACCC-3′; 5′-/56-FAM/CACAGGAGC/ZRN/CAAGAGTGAAGAACAGT/3IABkFQ/-3′
	PUM1	Pumilio RNA binding family member 1	NM_014676	5′-GAGCAGCAGAGATGTATCTTCC-3′; 5′-GACCAGGACATTCACAGACAC-3′; 5′-56-FAM/TCCTTCCCT/ZEN/CTCTTCACATGGATCCT/3IABkFQ/-3′
	RPLP0	Ribosomal protein lateral stalk subunit P0	NM_053275	5′-ACATCTCCCCCTTCTCCTT-3′; 5′-CAGACAGACACTGGCAACA-3′; 5′-/56-FAM/CCTGAAGTG/ZEN/CTTGATATCACAGAGGAAACT/3IAB kFQ/-3′

Table 1.
List of forward and reverse primers and probes used for qPCR (pre-designed and purchased from Integrated DNA Technologies (IDT)).

For differentiation experiments, aggregation of 5000 ASCs was induced as described above. After transferring to non-adhesive plates, the spheroids underwent induction of adipogenic differentiation in the same manner as the 2D cells. After 21 days of adipogenic differentiation, the spheroids were fixed 30 min with 4% PFA. After fixation, spheroids were washed 3× with PBS, followed by a 7 min incubation of 0.2% TritonX100 to permeabilize the cells for antibody penetration. To prevent non-specific binding, the spheroids were incubated in blocking buffer (0.1% BSA in PBS) for 30 min. The primary antibody (Perilipin-1 (D1D8) XP® Rabbit mAb, Cell Signaling Technologies; Danvers, MA, USA) was incubated at a 1:100 dilution overnight at 4°C. The secondary antibody (Alexa Fluor® 568 Donkey anti-rabbit IgG (H + L), Invitrogen) was incubated at 1:1000 for 30 min at room temperature. Between each step, cells were washed with PBS. As a last step, nuclear counterstaining was carried out by a 15 min incubation with the nuclear stain DAPI at room temperature, and then the spheroids were washed 2× with PBS, 1× with dH_2O, transferred onto glass slides and mounted with Glycergel (Dako; Carpinteria, CA, USA). The spheroids were analyzed on a confocal laser-scanning microscope (Axio ObserverZ1 attached to LSM700, Carl Zeiss, Göttingen, Germany; ×20 dry objective), using only the 568 nm excitation channel to document as many LDs as possible. Areas of the LDs were measured using ImageJ software (NIH, Maryland, USA).

2.8 Embedding of spheroids for semi-thin sectioning

Spheroids grown in hanging drops and differentiated as described above were fixed with half strength Karnovksy's fixative for 3 h. After 3× washing in 0.1 M cacodylate buffer at pH 7.4, samples were postfixed with 1% OsO_4 in cacodylate buffer for 3 h. Following 3× cacodylate buffer washing steps, spheroids were dehydrated by a graded series of ethanol with 3 changes of 100% ethanol and 2 subsequent changes of propylene oxide. Infiltration of epoxy resin Agar 100 (Science Services; Munich, Germany) were done in 3 ascending mixtures of propylene oxide/resin followed by incubation with pure resin overnight at 4°C. Samples were transferred into silicon molds with fresh resin and polymerized at 60°C for 2 days. Semithin sections (0.5 μm) were cut on a Reichert Ultracut™ S (Reichert, Austria) which were stained with Richardson's dye. Sections were analyzed and pictures were taken with Nikon microscope equipment (see above).

2.9 Preparation of histological sections and polarization microscopy

After biopsy, the tissues were cut into small pieces of about 3 mm^3 size and immediately fixed in 4% PFA.

After PFA fixation, the samples were processed by a conventional automated paraffin-embedding process (Leica, TP 1020 paraffin embedding processor). The samples were transferred to paraffin bloc molds. 5 μm sections were cut from the paraffin blocs. The tissue sections were subsequently "baked" for 2 h at 58°C. The sections were then deparaffinized using Rotihistol™ (Roth; Karlsruhe, Germany) and rehydrated in a series of ethanol solutions with lowering dilutions, washed with dH_2O and fixed with non-permanent CitiFluor™. The unstained sections were then imaged with a 10× objective on a light microscope with polarization filters (Axioplan, Carl Zeiss; Oberkochen, Germany) using the same wavelength for each image, captured with a digital camera (AxioCam, Carl Zeiss). The images were analyzed with ImageJ software.

Analysis included 6 biological repeats for lipedema and 3 biological repeats for control tissue.

2.10 Statistics

Statistical analyses were performed using GraphPad Prism software (version 9.0.0; La Jolla, CA, USA). Shapiro-Wilk tests were done to analyze if data were normally distributed. With data with normal distribution, Welch's t tests were performed. When the data were not normally distributed, Mann-Whitney tests were used.

3. Results and discussion

3.1 Lipogenesis and lipid droplets

In the present study, we have followed gene expression and in vitro growth of ASCs and fully differentiated adipocytes derived from the SVF of lipoaspirates from lipedema and control donors. Since we and others have shown previously that lipedema adipocytes differ from non-lipedema adipocytes by increased expression of adipogenesis-related genes (reviewed in [21, 22]), we went on to identify additional characteristics distinguishing lipedema adipocytes from their healthy counterparts.

Our gene expression study was performed using 2D cultures of lipedema and control adipocytes, while growth and LD size were studied in undifferentiated and differentiated 3D cultures generated by a conventional hanging drop method.

Here, we concentrated particularly on gene expression related to lipogenesis and the enlargement of LDs with a minor focus on inflammation and fibrosis-related gene expression. Furthermore, we addressed the question of whether the suggested hypertrophy of lipedema adipocytes described in vivo is also evident in a 3D test arrangement in vitro.

Interestingly, mRNA levels of alpha/beta hydrolase domain-containing protein 5 (ABHD5), a co-activator of adipose triglyceride lipase (ATGL) and key enzyme of cytosolic LD lipolysis [37] did not differ significantly between lipedema and non-lipedema adipocytes (**Figure 1**). ABHD5 plays a critical role in balancing basal and stimulated lipolysis. Under basal conditions, it stays bound to perilipin-1 (PLIN1) (described below), impeding its interaction with and activation of ATGL. Upon phosphorylation of PLIN1, ABHD5 dissociates from PLIN1 and interacts with ATGL, thereby activating the first and rate-limiting step in LD hydrolysis [38, 39]. Since ABHD5 expression was comparable in the lipedema and control group, we assume that under non-stimulated conditions, lipolysis in lipedema and non-lipedema cells is comparable, which was also reflected by the equal expression of ATGL (**Figure 1**).

We have demonstrated that mRNA levels of PLIN1 and the cell death-inducing DFFA-like effector protein C (CIDEC), also referred to as fat-specific protein 27 (FSP27), two proteins critically involved in the enlargement of LDs [40–42], are significantly upregulated in lipedema adipocytes compared to controls (**Figure 1**). PLIN1, a member of the PAT (perilipin, adipophilin, TIP47) family [43, 44], is robustly expressed in adipocytes of white and brown adipose tissue and associates physically with the surface of LDs. Its dual function is based on its ability to modulate lipid metabolism by blocking basal lipolysis but mediating hormone-stimulated hydrolysis of triacylglycerols [45–47]. PLIN1 binds to and activates CIDEC, a key component of LD fusion and enhancement of unilocular LDs in white adipocytes

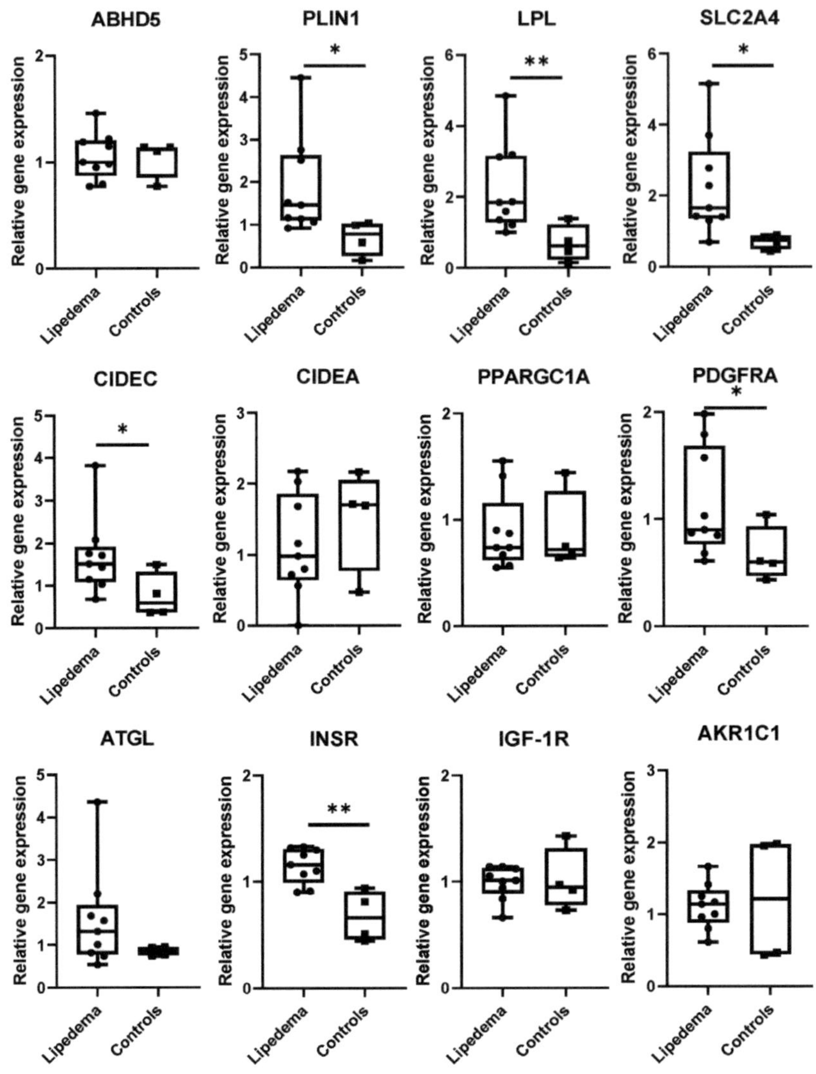

Figure 1.
*Relative gene expression after 21 days of adipogenic differentiation of lipedema (n = 9, BMI 26.7 ± 3.3 kg/m²) and controls (n = 4, BMI: 27.3 ± 3.2 kg/m²). *P < 0.05, **P < 0.01. Abbreviations: ABHD5: alpha/beta hydrolase domain-containing protein 5; PLIN1: Perilipin 1; LPL: lipoprotein lipase; SLC2A4: solute carrier family 2 member 4 gene, encoding the insulin-regulated glucose transporter GLUT4; CIDEC: cell death inducing DFFA like effector C (FSP27, fat-specific protein 27); CIDEA: cell death inducing DFFA like effector A; ATGL: adipose triglyceride lipase; PPARGC1A: peroxisome proliferator-activated receptor gamma coactivator 1-alpha; PDGFRA: platelet-derived growth factor receptor alpha; INSR: insulin receptor; IGF-1R: insulin-like growth factor 1 receptor; AKR1C1: aldo-keto reductase family 1 member C1.*

[40, 41]. CIDE proteins, currently comprising CIDEA, -B, and -C, localize at LD-LD contact sites and are involved in the directional lipid transfer between LDs, enabling LD fusion and enhancing lipid storage capacity of adipocytes [40].

As with all other members of the CIDE family, CIDEC was originally known for its apoptosis-promoting function in various cell types [48], but gradually emerged as major player in the regulation of lipolysis, storage of triglycerides and insulin signaling [49]. The antilipolytic activity of CIDEC is well documented [50]. It can directly interact with ATGL to inhibit its lipolytic activity, but may also engage in mediating the suppression of ATGL transcription [50]. Insulin significantly increases CIDEC mRNA levels, thereby facilitating the enlargement of LDs in adipocytes. This effect was abrogated upon depletion of CIDEC but not CIDEA [51].

It may be speculated that the upregulation of PLIN1 and CIDEC in lipedema adipocytes is indicative of LD enlargement contributing to the hypertrophy of lipedema adipose tissue.

We have shown that mRNA levels of the multifaceted lipoprotein lipase (LPL) and the insulin-related facilitative glucose transporter SLC2A4 (GLUT4), are significantly increased in lipedema adipocytes compared to controls (**Figure 1**), suggesting elevated lipogenesis and an overall increase in lipid turnover and metabolism [52, 53]. Upregulation of adipocyte LPL has also been linked to inflammation and macrophage activation in obese adipose tissue [54]. In addition, expression in preadipocytes was previously shown to correlate directly with increased intracellular lipid load [52]. This suggests that adipocyte-derived LPL is capable of managing efficient lipid storage in adipocytes without being dependent on extracellular, vascular-derived LPL activity. It will be interesting to clarify whether the adipocyte-intrinsic upregulation of LPL plays a role in lipedema adipose tissue hypertrophy.

Interestingly, mRNA levels of the insulin receptor (INSR) but not insulin-like growth factor-1 receptor (IGF-1R) are significantly elevated in lipedema adipocytes compared to controls. INSR and IGF-1R are highly homologous tyrosine kinase receptors with partly overlapping intracellular signaling pathways playing an essential role in adipose tissue development [55, 56]. However, despite their considerable structural and functional similarities, INSR and IGF-1R exert differential effects on white and brown adipose tissue differentiation [57]. As demonstrated in animal knockout experiments, development and maintenance of white adipose tissue is highly dependent on INSR while IGF-1R plays only a minor role in this respect [57]. Interestingly, INSR and IGF-1R are differentially expressed during adipogenic development. While IGF-1R levels exceed INSR levels in undifferentiated adipose cells, this situation is reversed in mature adipocytes [57, 58].

Although INSR and IGF-1R functions are primarily determined by ligand binding kinetics and intracellular tyrosine kinase activity, variations in mRNA levels could also contribute to alterations in insulin-induced cell response. In this respect, increased levels of INSR mRNA were observed in liver cells of genetically diabetic and obese mice [59]. Concerning the significantly increased expression of INSR mRNA in cultured lipedema adipocytes, additional studies are needed to determine whether this may impact insulin signaling and lipid metabolism in lipedema adipose tissue.

Results from our molecular study further reveal that platelet-derived growth factor receptor-alpha (PDGFRA) mRNA levels are significantly increased in lipedema adipocytes compared to controls. Of note, PDGFRA was shown to play a crucial role in adipose organogenesis by controlling the adipogenic and fibrogenic differentiation of precursor cells [60, 61]. Although further in-depth studies are still missing, it cannot be ruled out that PDGFRA plays a role in the development of lipedema-associated fibrosis.

Neither aldo-keto reductase 1C1 (AKR1C1), a gene involved in progesterone metabolism and upregulated in a family with non-syndromic lipedema [62], nor the peroxisome proliferator-activated receptor gamma coactivator 1-alpha (PPARGC1A), a key regulator of energy metabolism, glucose uptake and mitochondrial biogenesis [63] showed differential expression in lipedema and non-lipedema adipocytes.

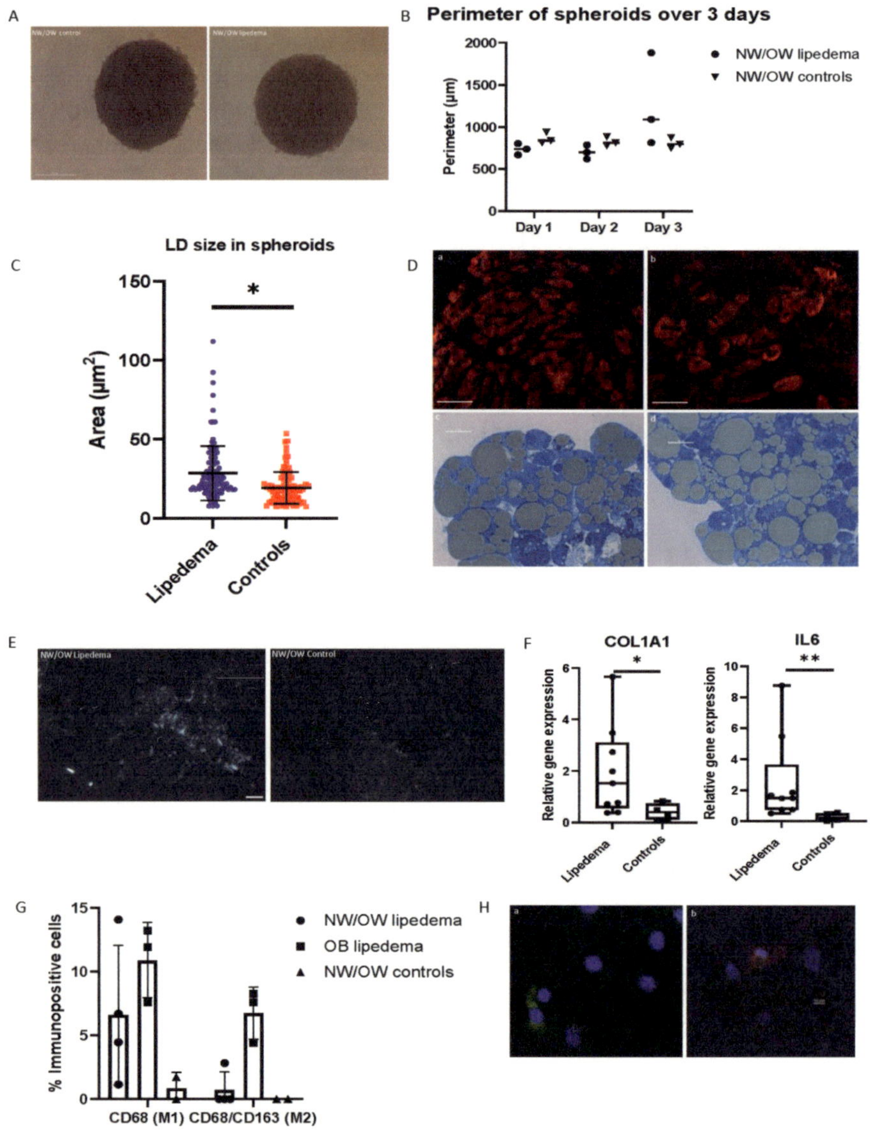

Figure 2.

*(A) Morphological analysis of spheroids grown from lipedema and control ASCs. Scale bar: 200 µm. (B) Perimeter was measured using ImageJ software (NIH, Maryland, USA) in NW/OW lipedema (n = 3, BMI = 21.7 ± 0.4 kg/m²) and controls (n = 3, BMI = 25.7 ± 2.5 kg/m²). NW/OW: normal weight/overweight. (C) Size of lipid droplets (LD) measured in in vitro differentiated spheroids grown from lipedema and control ASCs. NW/OW lipedema (n = 3, BMI = 23.7 ± 1.4 kg/m²), NW/OW controls (n = 3, BMI = 24.3 ± 0.4 kg/m²). (*P < 0.05). (D) Representative images of PLIN1 expression in lipedema (a) and control (b) spheroids, scale bar: 100 µm, and semi-thin sections of in vitro differentiated lipedema (c) and control (d) spheroids, scale bar: 10 µm. PLIN1: Perilipin-1. (E) Representative polarization microscopy images of biopsied lipedema and control subcutaneous adipose tissue from lateral thighs of lipedema and control donors (both BMI 24.0 kg/m²). Scale bar: 100 µm. (F) Relative gene expression of collagen 1 (COL1A1) and interleukin-6 (IL6) in adipocytes after 21 days of adipogenic differentiation. Lipedema (n = 9, BMI 26.7 ± 3.3 kg/m²). Controls (n = 4, BMI = 27.3 ± 3.2 kg/m²). Comparison of COL1A1: *P < 0.05. Comparison of IL6: **P < 0.01. G) Quantitative evaluation of M1 and M2 macrophage abundance in lipedema NW/OW (n = 4, BMI = 22.8 ± 1.0 kg/m²), lipedema OB (n = 3, BMI = 39.4 ± 2.1 kg/m²) and control (n = 2, BMI = 24.3 ± 0.5 kg/m²) cultures. NW/OW: normal weight/overweight; OB: obese. Co-expression of CD68 and CD163 is predominantly found in ASCs from obese donors. (H) Immunoreactivity of (a) CD68 and (b) CD68/CD163 positive cells in lipedema ASC cultures. Representative examples are shown.*

3.2 Growth and hypertrophy of 3D ASC and adipocyte cultures

In this set of experiments, we focused on the growth of spheroids originating from SVF/ASCs from NW/OW and OB lipedema donors compared to controls. No significant difference in growth and morphology was detectable between 3D aggregates grown from lipedema and control ASCs, while a slight increase in the perimeters of spheroids from lipedema ASCs was observed after 3 days of cultivation, **Figure 2A** and **B**.

Next, we addressed the question whether LDs of in vitro-differentiated adipocytes grown in 3D cultures differ in size between lipedema and control cells. Our results show that the average size of LDs is significantly increased in lipedema spheroids compared to controls (**Figure 2C**). This supports earlier findings demonstrating increased hypertrophy of adipocytes in normal weight lipedema adipose tissue compared to BMI-matched controls [18, 30, 35, 36]. Interestingly, LDs in lipedema spheroids showed a more heterogeneous picture and contained a higher number of disproportionately large droplets compared to controls (**Figure 2D**).

3.3 Fibrosis- and inflammation-associated markers

As evidenced by our gene expression studies, augmented deposition of collagen was detectable in histological sections from biopsied subcutaneous adipose tissue from women with lipedema compared to controls (**Figure 2E**). In line with this, lipedema adipocytes differ from controls by their significantly increased expression of collagen 1 (COL1A1) and interleukin-6 (IL-6) mRNA (**Figure 2F**), emphasizing again the inflammatory and fibrotic component of lipedema pathology.

Our results from immunostainings reveal elevated numbers of M1 macrophages (evidenced by a granulated signal) in lipedema ASCs compared to controls (**Figure 2G** and **H**). This confirms earlier reports, demonstrating increased immune cell infiltration into lipedema adipose tissue [30, 32, 35, 36, 64–66]. In our study, only low numbers of activated (M2) macrophages, characterized by the selective marker CD163 with additional expression of CD68 were present in lipedema cultured cells, while the highest percentage of M2 macrophages was detected in ASCs from OB donors. Control ASCs were devoid of activated (M2) macrophages. Again, this confirms the general notion that excessive weight gain triggers inflammatory and fibrotic mechanisms, especially in lipedema.

4. Conclusion

The significantly increased transcriptional upregulation of genes involved in the regulation of LD growth distinguishes in vitro differentiated lipedema adipocytes from their healthy counterparts. Although further experimental evidence is needed it may be speculated that the hypertrophic nature of lipedema tissue may be maintained in vitro throughout cultivation.

Increased expression of INSR, GLUT4, and LPL in lipedema adipocytes suggests involvement of insulin signaling in lipedema adipose hypertrophy.

In addition, our data support the notion that lipedema pathogenesis is accompanied by inflammatory and fibrotic conditions. Concerning lipedema-associated fibrosis, the upregulation of PDGFRA might open a new field of research, focusing on a potential imbalance of adipogenic and stromal differentiation at early stages of lipedema development. Thus, future research should concentrate on the initial stages of lipedema, when the earliest signs of adipose tissue alterations appear, and inflammation-related changes are not yet prevalent.

Acknowledgements

This work was supported by the Land Salzburg (project number 20204-WISS/240/3-2019). We thank H. Tempfer (Paracelsus Medical University of Salzburg) for valuable assistance with confocal microscopy. Dr. C. Giera (LipoClinic Dr. Heck) and Dres N. Broer and P. Heidekrueger (LIPOhelp, Salzburg) are gratefully acknowledged for providing adipose tissue samples.

Author details

Anna Maria Ernst[1*], Erwin Schimak[1], Marianne Steiner[1], Anna-Theresa Lipp[2], Hans-Christian Bauer[1,3,4] and Hannelore Bauer[1*]

1 Department of Biosciences, Paris Lodron University of Salzburg, Salzburg, Austria

2 PANTEA Private Clinic, Munich, Germany

3 Institute of Tendon and Bone Regeneration, Spinal Cord Injury and Tissue Regeneration Center, Paracelsus Medical University, Salzburg, Austria

4 Austrian Cluster for Tissue Regeneration, Vienna, Austria

*Address all correspondence to: anna_maria.ernst@stud.plus.ac.at and hannelore.bauer@plus.ac.at

IntechOpen

© 2024 The Author(s). Licensee IntechOpen. This chapter is distributed under the terms of the Creative Commons Attribution License (http://creativecommons.org/licenses/by/3.0), which permits unrestricted use, distribution, and reproduction in any medium, provided the original work is properly cited.

References

[1] Buck DW 2nd, Herbst KL. Lipedema: A relatively common disease with extremely common misconceptions. Plastic and Reconstructive Surgery Global Open. 2016;**4**(9):e1043

[2] Kruppa P, Georgiou I, Biermann N, Prantl L, Klein-Weigel P, Ghods M. Lipedema-pathogenesis, diagnosis, and treatment options. Deutsches Ärzteblatt International. 2020;**117**(22-23):396-403

[3] Okhovat JP, Alavi A. Lipedema: A review of the literature. The International journal of Lower Extremity Wounds. 2015;**14**(3):262-267

[4] Vyas A, Adnan G. Lipedema. In: StatPearls. Treasure Island (FL) Companies: StatPearls Publishing LLC; 2023

[5] Wollina U. Lipedema-An update. Dermatologic Therapy. 2019;**32**(2):e12805

[6] Torre YS, Wadeea R, Rosas V, Herbst KL. Lipedema: Friend and foe. Hormone Molecular Biology and Clinical Investigation. 2018;**33**(1):20170076

[7] Child AH, Gordon KD, Sharpe P, Brice G, Ostergaard P, Jeffery S, et al. Lipedema: An inherited condition. American Journal of Medical Genetics Part A. 2010;**152a**(4):970-976

[8] Paolacci S, Precone V, Acquaviva F, Chiurazzi P, Fulcheri E, Pinelli M, et al. Genetics of lipedema: New perspectives on genetic research and molecular diagnoses. European Review for Medical and Pharmacological Sciences. 2019;**23**(13):5581-5594

[9] Forner-Cordero I, Forner-Cordero A, Szolnoky G. Update in the management of lipedema. International Angiology. 2021;**40**(4):345-357

[10] Bauer AT, von Lukowicz D, Lossagk K, Aitzetmueller M, Moog P, Cerny M, et al. New insights on lipedema: The Enigmatic disease of the peripheral fat. Plastic and Reconstructive Surgery. 2019;**144**(6):1475-1484

[11] Katzer K, Hill JL, McIver KB, Foster MT. Lipedema and the potential role of estrogen in excessive adipose tissue accumulation. International Journal of Molecular Sciences. 2021;**22**(21):11720

[12] Herbst KL. Subcutaneous adipose tissue diseases: Dercum disease, lipedema, familial multiple lipomatosis, and madelung disease. In: Feingold KR, Anawalt B, Blackman MR, Boyce A, Chrousos G, Corpas E, et al., editors. Endotext. South Dartmouth (MA): MDText.com, Inc. Copyright © 2000-2023, MDText.com, Inc.; 2000

[13] Földi M, Földi E. Földi's Textbook of Lymphology: For Physicians and Lymphedema Therapists. 3rd ed. Germany: Mosby, Elsevier; 2006. pp. 417-427

[14] Reich-Schupke S, Schmeller W, Brauer WJ, Cornely ME, Faerber G, Ludwig M, et al. S1 guidelines: Lipedema. Journal der Deutschen Dermatologischen Gesellschaft = Journal of the German Society of Dermatology: JDDG. 2017;**15**(7):758-767

[15] Duhon BH, Phan TT, Taylor SL, Crescenzi RL, Rutkowski JM. Current mechanistic understandings of lymphedema and lipedema: Tales of fluid, fat, and fibrosis. International Journal of Molecular Sciences. 2022;**23**(12):6621

[16] Shavit E, Wollina U, Alavi A. Lipoedema is not lymphoedema: A review of current literature. International Wound Journal. 2018;**15**(6):921-928

[17] Pereira de Godoy LM, Pereira de Godoy HJ, de Godoy P, Capeletto P, Guerreiro Godoy MF, Pereira de Godoy JM. Lipedema and the evolution to lymphedema with the progression of obesity. Cureus. 2020;**12**(12):e11854

[18] von Atzigen J, Burger A, Grünherz L, Barbon C, Felmerer G, Giovanoli P, et al. A comparative analysis to dissect the histological and molecular differences among lipedema, lipohypertrophy and secondary lymphedema. International Journal of Molecular Sciences. 2023;**24**(8):7591

[19] Wold LE, Hines EA Jr, Allen EV. Lipedema of the legs; a syndrome characterized by fat legs and edema. Annals of Internal Medicine. 1951;**34**(5):1243-1250

[20] Bertsch T, Erbacher G, Elwell R. Lipoedema: A paradigm shift and consensus. Journal of Wound Care. 2020;**29**(Sup11b):1-51

[21] Ernst AM, Bauer H, Bauer HC, Steiner M, Malfertheiner A, Lipp AT. Lipedema research-quo vadis? Journal of Personalized Medicine. 2022;13(1):98

[22] Poojari A, Dev K, Rabiee A. Lipedema: Insights into morphology, pathophysiology, and challenges. Biomedicine. 2022;**10**(12):3081

[23] Peprah K, MacDougall D. CADTH Rapid Response Reports. Liposuction for the Treatment of Lipedema: A Review of Clinical Effectiveness and Guidelines. Ottawa (ON): Canadian Agency for Drugs and Technologies in Health Copyright © 2019 Canadian Agency for Drugs and Technologies in Health; 2019

[24] Herbst KL. Rare adipose disorders (RADs) masquerading as obesity. Acta Pharmacologica Sinica. 2012;**33**(2):155-172

[25] Amato ACM, Saucedo DZ, Santos KDS, Benitti DA. Ultrasound criteria for lipedema diagnosis. Phlebology. 2021;**36**(8):651-658

[26] Clarke C, Kirby JN, Smidt T, Best T. Stages of lipoedema: Experiences of physical and mental health and health care. Quality of Life Research. 2023;**32**(1):127-137

[27] Jo J, Gavrilova O, Pack S, Jou W, Mullen S, Sumner AE, et al. Hypertrophy and/or hyperplasia: Dynamics of adipose tissue growth. PLoS Computational Biology. 2009;**5**(3):e1000324

[28] Hepler C, Gupta RK. The expanding problem of adipose depot remodeling and postnatal adipocyte progenitor recruitment. Molecular and Cellular Endocrinology. 2017;**445**:95-108

[29] Kruppa P, Gohlke S, Łapiński K, Garcia-Carrizo F, Soultoukis GA, Infanger M, et al. Lipedema stage affects adipocyte hypertrophy, subcutaneous adipose tissue inflammation and interstitial fibrosis. Frontiers in Immunology. 2023;**14**:1223264

[30] Felmerer G, Stylianaki A, Hägerling R, Wang A, Ströbel P, Hollmén M, et al. Adipose tissue hypertrophy, an aberrant biochemical profile and distinct gene expression in lipedema. The Journal of Surgical Research. 2020;**253**:294-303

[31] Ishaq M, Bandara N, Morgan S, Nowell C, Mehdi AM, Lyu R, et al. Key signaling networks are dysregulated in patients with the adipose tissue disorder, lipedema. International Journal of Obesity. 2022;**46**(3):502-514

[32] Priglinger E, Wurzer C, Steffenhagen C, Maier J, Hofer V, Peterbauer A, et al. The adipose tissue-derived stromal vascular fraction cells from lipedema patients: Are they different? Cytotherapy. 2017;**19**(7):849-860

[33] Bauer AT, von Lukowicz D, Lossagk K, Hopfner U, Kirsch M, Moog P, et al. adipose stem cells from lipedema and control adipose tissue respond differently to adipogenic stimulation in vitro. Plastic and Reconstructive Surgery. 2019;**144**(3):623-632

[34] Al-Ghadban S, Diaz ZT, Singer HJ, Mert KB, Bunnell BA. Increase in leptin and PPAR-γ gene expression in lipedema adipocytes differentiated in vitro from adipose-derived stem cells. Cell. 2020;**9**(2):430

[35] Al-Ghadban S, Cromer W, Allen M, Ussery C, Badowski M, Harris D, et al. Dilated blood and lymphatic microvessels, angiogenesis, increased macrophages, and adipocyte hypertrophy in lipedema thigh skin and fat tissue. Journal of Obesity. 2019;**2019**:8747461

[36] Wolf S, Deuel JW, Hollmén M, Felmerer G, Kim BS, Vasella M, et al. A distinct cytokine profile and stromal vascular fraction metabolic status without significant changes in the lipid composition characterizes lipedema. International Journal of Molecular Sciences. 2021;**22**(7):3313

[37] Yu L, Li Y, Grisé A, Wang H. CGI-58: Versatile regulator of intracellular lipid droplet homeostasis. Advances in Experimental Medicine and Biology. 2020;**1276**:197-222

[38] Lass A, Zimmermann R, Haemmerle G, Riederer M, Schoiswohl G, Schweiger M, et al. Adipose triglyceride lipase-mediated lipolysis of cellular fat stores is activated by CGI-58 and defective in Chanarin-Dorfman Syndrome. Cell Metabolism. 2006;**3**(5):309-319

[39] Zimmermann R, Strauss JG, Haemmerle G, Schoiswohl G, Birner-Gruenberger R, Riederer M, et al. Fat mobilization in adipose tissue is promoted by adipose triglyceride lipase. Science. 2004;**306**(5700):1383-1386

[40] Chen FJ, Yin Y, Chua BT, Li P. CIDE family proteins control lipid homeostasis and the development of metabolic diseases. Traffic. 2020;**21**(1):94-105

[41] Gao G, Chen FJ, Zhou L, Su L, Xu D, Xu L, et al. Control of lipid droplet fusion and growth by CIDE family proteins. Biochimica et Biophysica Acta - Molecular and Cell Biology of Lipids. 2017;**1862**(10 Pt B):1197-1204

[42] Olzmann JA, Carvalho P. Dynamics and functions of lipid droplets. Nature Reviews. Molecular Cell Biology. 2019;**20**(3):137-155

[43] Bickel PE, Tansey JT, Welte MA. PAT proteins, an ancient family of lipid droplet proteins that regulate cellular lipid stores. Biochimica et Biophysica Acta. 2009;**1791**(6):419-440

[44] Kimmel AR, Brasaemle DL, McAndrews-Hill M, Sztalryd C, Londos C. Adoption of PERILIPIN as a unifying nomenclature for the mammalian PAT-family of intracellular lipid storage droplet proteins. Journal of Lipid Research. 2010;**51**(3):468-471

[45] Londos C, Sztalryd C, Tansey JT, Kimmel AR. Role of PAT proteins in lipid metabolism. Biochimie. 2005;**87**(1):45-49

[46] Kimmel AR, Sztalryd C. The perilipins: Major cytosolic lipid droplet-associated proteins and their roles in

cellular lipid storage, mobilization, and systemic homeostasis. Annual Review of Nutrition. 2016;**36**:471-509

[47] Miyoshi H, Souza SC, Zhang HH, Strissel KJ, Christoffolete MA, Kovsan J, et al. Perilipin promotes hormone-sensitive lipase-mediated adipocyte lipolysis via phosphorylation-dependent and -independent mechanisms. The Journal of Biological Chemistry. 2006;**281**(23):15837-15844

[48] Yonezawa T, Kurata R, Kimura M, Inoko H. Which CIDE are you on? Apoptosis and energy metabolism. Molecular BioSystems. 2011;**7**(1):91-100

[49] Grahn THM, Kaur R, Yin J, Schweiger M, Sharma VM, Lee MJ, et al. Fat-specific protein 27 (FSP27) interacts with adipose triglyceride lipase (ATGL) to regulate lipolysis and insulin sensitivity in human adipocytes. The Journal of Biological Chemistry. 2014;**289**(17):12029-12039

[50] Singh M, Kaur R, Lee MJ, Pickering RT, Sharma VM, Puri V, et al. Fat-specific protein 27 inhibits lipolysis by facilitating the inhibitory effect of transcription factor Egr1 on transcription of adipose triglyceride lipase. The Journal of Biological Chemistry. 2014;**289**(21):14481-14487

[51] Ito M, Nagasawa M, Hara T, Ide T, Murakami K. Differential roles of CIDEA and CIDEC in insulin-induced anti-apoptosis and lipid droplet formation in human adipocytes. Journal of Lipid Research. 2010;**51**(7):1676-1684

[52] Gonzales AM, Orlando RA. Role of adipocyte-derived lipoprotein lipase in adipocyte hypertrophy. Nutrition & Metabolism (London). 2007;**4**:22

[53] Mead JR, Irvine SA, Ramji DP. Lipoprotein lipase: Structure, function, regulation, and role in disease. Journal of Molecular Medicine (Berlin, Germany). 2002;**80**(12):753-769

[54] Li L, Renier G. Adipocyte-derived lipoprotein lipase induces macrophage activation and monocyte adhesion: Role of fatty acids. Obesity (Silver Spring, Md). 2007;**15**(11):2595-2604

[55] Haeusler RA, McGraw TE, Accili D. Biochemical and cellular properties of insulin receptor signalling. Nature Reviews. Molecular Cell Biology. 2018;**19**(1):31-44

[56] Hakuno F, Takahashi SI. IGF1 receptor signaling pathways. Journal of Molecular Endocrinology. 2018;**61**(1):T69-t86

[57] Boucher J, Softic S, El Ouaamari A, Krumpoch MT, Kleinridders A, Kulkarni RN, et al. Differential roles of insulin and IGF-1 receptors in adipose tissue development and function. Diabetes. 2016;**65**(8): 2201-2213

[58] Entingh-Pearsall A, Kahn CR. Differential roles of the insulin and insulin-like growth factor-I (IGF-I) receptors in response to insulin and IGF-I. The Journal of Biological Chemistry. 2004;**279**(36):38016-38024

[59] Ludwig S, Muller-Wieland D, Goldstein BJ, Kahn CR. The insulin receptor gene and its expression in insulin-resistant mice. Endocrinology. 1988;**123**(1):594-600

[60] Shin S, Pang Y, Park J, Liu L, Lukas BE, Kim SH, et al. Dynamic control of adipose tissue development and adult tissue homeostasis by platelet-derived growth factor receptor alpha. eLife. 2020;**9**:e56189

[61] Marcelin G, Ferreira A, Liu Y, Atlan M, Aron-Wisnewsky J, Pelloux V,

et al. A PDGFRα-mediated switch toward CD9(high) adipocyte progenitors controls obesity-induced adipose tissue fibrosis. Cell Metabolism. 2017;**25**(3):673-685

[62] Michelini S, Chiurazzi P, Marino V, Dell'Orco D, Manara E, Baglivo M, et al. Aldo-Keto Reductase 1C1 (AKR1C1) as the first mutated gene in a family with nonsyndromic primary lipedema. International Journal of Molecular Sciences. 2020;**21**(17):6264

[63] Tiraby C, Langin D. PGC-1alpha, a transcriptional coactivator involved in metabolism. Medical Science (Paris). 2005;**21**(1):49-54

[64] Strohmeier K, Hofmann M, Jacak J, Narzt MS, Wahlmueller M, Mairhofer M, et al. Multi-level analysis of adipose tissue reveals the relevance of perivascular subpopulations and an increased endothelial permeability in early-stage lipedema. Biomedicine. 2022;**10**(5):1163

[65] Suga H, Araki J, Aoi N, Kato H, Higashino T, Yoshimura K. Adipose tissue remodeling in lipedema: Adipocyte death and concurrent regeneration. Journal of Cutaneous Pathology. 2009;**36**(12):1293-1298

[66] Wolf S, Rannikko JH, Virtakoivu R, Cinelli P, Felmerer G, Burger A, et al. A distinct M2 macrophage infiltrate and transcriptomic profile decisively influence adipocyte differentiation in lipedema. Frontiers in Immunology. 2022;**13**:1004609

Section 3

Brown Adipose Tissue Homeostasis in Health and Disease

Chapter 5

Brown and Beige Adipose Tissue: From Activators to Physiological Relevance

Dominik Tischer and Ana Soriano-Arroquia

Abstract

Brown and beige adipose tissue activate non-shivering thermogenesis in response to cold exposure or beta-adrenergic agonists. During this process, glucose and lipids are used to generate heat through mitochondrial uncoupling, increasing energy expenditure at the expense of adenosine triphosphate (ATP) production. Importantly, the decline in brown adipose tissue negatively correlates with age and body mass index (BMI). This is, therefore, why induced "browning" of white adipose tissue is proposed as a promising therapeutic approach against obesity and metabolic diseases. In this chapter, we will review the intricate and exciting world of non-shivering thermogenesis, from the molecular mechanisms to the potential pharmacological treatments that are currently under scientific scrutiny, as well as the role that batokines, BAT-derived adipokines, play in inter-tissue crosstalk after certain stimuli such as cold exposure and exercise.

Keywords: brown and beige adipose tissue, BAT, browning, cold exposure, exercise, Ucp1

1. Introduction

Brown and beige adipose tissues play a critical role in maintaining whole body core temperature as a protective mechanism against cold stressors. Unlike white adipose tissue, thermogenic adipose tissue is specialized in producing heat by using glucose and fatty acids as substrates. The heat generated during non-shivering thermogenesis is the result of protons pumped back into the mitochondrial matrix from the intermembrane space during oxidative phosphorylation by an uncoupler protein or chemical, bypassing ATP synthase, which results in increased energy expenditure that can be directly measured by heat loss. This process is crucial in maintaining body temperature, particularly in cold environments, and serves as a natural way for the body to regulate energy balance.

An important aspect of brown adipose tissue (BAT) function is its decline with advancing age and increasing BMI. Studies have shown that, as individuals age or become overweight, the amount and activity of brown fat decrease significantly. This decline is associated with a reduced ability to undergo non-shivering thermogenesis, which in turn may contribute to the development of metabolic disorders, including obesity and type-2 diabetes. Consequently, the search for ways to activate or increase the amount of brown and beige adipose tissue has become an exciting area of research, particularly in the context of therapeutic interventions for obesity and metabolic diseases.

One of the most promising strategies currently being explored is the concept of "browning" white adipose tissue. This refers to the process by which white adipocytes, which typically store energy, are induced to adopt characteristics similar to brown adipocytes, thereby acquiring the ability to burn energy and generate heat. The induction of browning in white adipose tissue is seen as a potential therapeutic approach for combating obesity, as it could help to increase energy expenditure in individuals with excess body fat. Numerous pharmacological and lifestyle interventions, such as cold exposure, exercise and certain dietary components, have been shown to promote the browning of white adipose tissue, and these approaches are the subject of intense scientific investigation.

In this chapter, we will delve into the fascinating and complex world of non-shivering thermogenesis, exploring not only the molecular mechanisms that underlie this process but also the various ways in which it can be modulated for therapeutic purposes. We will review current research on potential pharmacological treatments aimed at enhancing brown and beige fat activity, including the use of beta-adrenergic agonists and other agents that target biological pathways regulating mitochondrial uncoupling.

By the end of this chapter, we aim to provide a comprehensive overview of the current understanding of non-shivering thermogenesis, from the basic biological mechanisms to the therapeutic possibilities that are being explored in clinical and preclinical settings. Understanding how brown and beige adipose tissues contribute to energy balance and metabolic health could open up new avenues for the treatment of obesity and related metabolic diseases, offering hope for interventions that harness the body's natural thermogenic processes to promote better health outcomes.

2. Brown adipose tissue physiology and functionality

2.1 BAT localization and physiology

The adipose tissue is composed of white, brown or pink (in females) multi-located fat depots across the whole organism [1]. Anatomical compositions of the pads composing the different depots are found between humans and mice. In both species, the main depots of white adipose tissue (WAT) represent areas underneath the skin (subcutaneous) and surrounding the viscera (visceral depots). In mice and human infants, BAT is mainly located in the interscapular and perirenal regions. In the adult humans, BAT is mainly found in the supraclavicular region, but also in the cervical, paravertebral, axillary and periaortic areas (**Tables 1** and **2**) [2].

There are major differences between white and brown adipocytes. Brown adipocytes are cells with multilocular lipid droplets, a central nucleus and a cytoplasm highly enriched in mitochondria and characterized by the expression of the uncoupled protein UCP1. On the other side, white adipocytes present an unilocular lipid droplet, less mitochondria content and a nucleus located in the periphery. In addition, BAT is highly vascularized while white adipose tissue present low vascularization [1].

Alternatively, we can also find another type of adipocyte that belongs to an intermediate phenotype between brown and white: the beige or brite adipocytes. Beige

Humans	Model in mice
Visceral WAT (VAT)	Gonadal (epididymal) depots of WAT around testes/ovaries
Subcutaneous WAT (SAT) →*greater propensity of browning*	Inguinal subcutaneous depots in the anterior and upper hind limbs →*greater propensity of browning*

Table 1.
Main locations of white adipose tissue (WAT) in humans and the corresponding depots used in murine models based on Ref. [2].

	Mouse	Human
Location	BAT is largely located in the interscapular region, but also in the cervical, axillary, pariaortic, perireral and paravertebral regions. Supraclavicular BAT has also been described.	BAT is largely located in the supraclavicular region, but also in the cervical, axillary, periaortic, paravertebral and perirenal regions. Interscapular (human babies, disappears during adolescence)
Measurement	• Indirect calorimetry: Gas exchange in terms of oxygen consumed (O_2) versus carbon dioxide produced (CO_2) is used to calculate energy expenditure (EE). • Maximal thermogenic capacity: BAT is stimulated with a β3-adrenergic receptor agonist such as CL (CL316243) after acclimatization at thermoneutrality or cold exposure. Energy expenditure is measured by indirect calorimetry.	• Indirect calorimetry • Positron emission tomography coupled with computed tomography (PET/CT) during infusion of radiolabeled 18-fluorodeoxyglucose (^{18}F-FDG); measures glucose uptake in BAT after cold or β3-adrenergic receptor agonist (e.g., Mirabegron) • Magnetic resonance (MRI) • Single photon emission-computed tomography (SPECT) • Ultrasound • Infrared imaging • Circulating biomarkers

Table 2.
Main locations of brown adipose tissue in humans and mice and the most common approaches used for the localization and measurement of BAT activity based on Refs. [2, 3].

adipocytes are a heterogeneous population of cells with thermogenic capacity that are present in WAT depots. This thermogenic capacity is reversible, that is, specific responses to the environment will determine whether there is white-to-beige or beige-to-white trans-differentiation, highlighting the huge plasticity and clinical potential of WAT [1, 4]. The fact that brown and beige adipose depots cannot be distinguishable using ^{18}F-FDG-PET/CT in humans has led to the interchangeable use of both terms when referring to adult individuals. Yet, distinct cellular lineages will rise to either brown or beige/white adipocytes: both beige and white adipocytes derived from Myf5 negative adipose-derived mesenchymal stem cells (AMSCs). Brown adipocytes precursors, contrarily, express myogenic markers such as Myf5, revealing a transcriptional signature overlap between both skeletal muscle and BAT [5]. In fact, loss of expression of positive regulatory domain containing 16 (PRDM16) stimulates the differentiation of brown adipocytes into muscle cells, while myoblasts differentiate into brown adipocytes when PRDM16 is ectopically increased, a process mediated by the co-activation of the peroxisome proliferator-activated receptor gamma (PPAR-γ) [6, 7].

The most important locations and different depots of beige adipose and BAT are classified below:

- Mice and infants: interscapular region
- Adult humans: supraclavicular/mediastinal
- Adipocytes in interscapular BAT from infants are characteristic of classical brown adipocytes.
- Adipocytes in BAT depots from adults are a mixed population of UCP1 positive and negative cells
- Beige cells from inguinal WAT (iWAT): conversion of white adipocytes by a process known as demasking or trans-differentiation
- Beige cells from gonadal/epididymal WAT (gWAT): newly differentiated from progenitor cells (CD34, SCA1, PDGFRα)

2.2 Significance of brown adipose tissue in the adult human

BAT is known as the master regulator of non-shivering thermogenesis under cold stress, particularly in infants who lack the capability to shiver [8]. It was initially thought that BAT mass and activity progressively declined to undetectable levels during the adulthood. However, the introduction of 18-fluor-deoxyglucose (^{18}F-FDG) positron emission tomography (PET) and computed tomography (CT) technologies in the twenty-first century allowed the detection of BAT also in adult individuals [9–12].

Even though there is an increase of adiposity with age, particularly of white adipose tissue, it was discovered that active beige and BAT (BAT) declines during aging and inversely correlates with BMI and blood glucose levels. In turn, higher presence of BAT in humans is associated with leanness, lower prevalence of cardiovascular disease, and generally improved metabolic health [13–16]. One of these studies was performed by Tobias Becher et al. published in Nature Medicine Letters in 2021, where they retrospectively analyzed ^{18}F-FDG PET/CT scans from 52,487 patients initially performed for the diagnosis or treatment of cancer. The scans revealed that BAT presence correlates with:

- Lower prevalence of cardiovascular diseases
- Improved blood glucose
- Beneficial effects are more pronounced in patients with obesity
- Inversely correlates with ambient temperature, BMI and glucose levels
- Decreases with age
- More prevalent in women

From all the patients, BAT was reported in only 9.7% of the individuals, and it negatively correlated to the use of statins and beta-blockers. Of note, BAT also showed a direct correlation with the site of the tumor, particularly in some types of cancer, such as oral and breast cancer [13]. These findings were in consonance with previous studies that already found a relationship between BAT activity and cancer. For example, an earlier retrospective analysis revealed that BAT was higher, particularly in younger women with breast cancer compared to the control group. However, no significant differences were found between women who were more than 55 years old [17].

Interestingly, a more recent study in Nature claims that cold-induced activation of BAT promotes starvation of the tumor micro-environment in several murine models of cancer, decreasing the size of the tumor and increasing the survival of the mice [18]. This effect is achieved by mutual competition between BAT and the tumor for circulating glucose. After cold, glucose uptake is prioritized in BAT, limiting its supply to the tumor and forcing cancer cells to metabolically shift from aerobic glycolysis (also known as Warburg effect) to oxidative phosphorylation [18].

2.3 The high adaptability of BAT: The real contribution to energy expenditure

BAT has been hypothesized to present high plasticity and adaptability to diverse circumstances and environments. In fact, the type and intensity of the stimuli (e.g., cold) that activates the tissue is as important as the timing and duration of such stressors. This will determine whether the associated changes are either acute responses to maintain physiological balance or homeostasis or whether acclimatization or even non-reversible genetic changes via natural selection pursued along generations in response to long-term adaptations to a specific environment [19].

In mammals, and generally in endothermic animals, the range of temperature where the body can maintain the core temperature through metabolic activity without the use of physical activity (i.e., at rest) and during fasting is known as the thermoneutral zone, when the production of heat as byproduct of metabolism balance the loss of "dry" heat from the epidermis to the environment, a process achieved by increased blood flow through the circulatory system. This concept is characterized by the basal metabolic rate (BMR), which is the minimum energy required needed to maintain vital functions at rest [20].

When the environmental temperature decreases, heat generation is enhanced to maintain core body temperature. Initially, this is accomplished through shivering thermogenesis by the skeletal muscle. However, when cold is sustained during a prolonged period of time, the organism adapts to the new environment by notably increasing blood flow to the BAT. This observation was accompanied by a slight increase in blood flow also to the skeletal muscle and at the expense of shivering, first defined in rats by Foster and Frydman in 1978 [21]. The discovery strengthens the hypothesis of BAT as the major contributor to non-shivering thermogenesis despite its small size (at least 60% versus 12% of the calorigenic response to cold acclimatation by the skeletal muscle).

In humans, prolonged fasting to mimic insulin-resistance conditions in healthy individuals, glucose uptake and non-shivering thermogenesis are decreased in BAT under cold stimulation, while other thermogenic tissues such as white adipose tissue and skeletal muscle are not affected. Reduced glucose uptake by BAT was accompanied by lower core temperature, emphasizing again the important role of BAT in maintaining body temperature during cold. However, this study unveils the question of whether the skeletal muscle or white adipose tissue might be more prominent therapeutic targets to boost glucose clearance through cold exposure under insulin-resistance conditions such as type-2 diabetes [22].

Yet, the total contribution of BAT in energy expenditure and the plausible role of the skeletal muscle is still controversial for some scientists. For instance, Carpentier and Blondin critically challenge the assumption that activation of BAT in humans has a real therapeutic effect. To date, the use of 18 F-fluoro-deoxyglocose (^{18}F-FDG) PET, in combination with magnetic resonance imaging (MRI) or CT, is the gold standard method to identify BAT location and glucose uptake. This has been an indisputable useful technology that allowed for the assessment of BAT volume and metabolic function in humans. However, many concerns arise since ^{18}F-FDG PET assumes glucose as a sole fuel of energy and neglects other plausible sources, such as circulating fatty acids [23]. Of note, Carpentier and Blondin highlighted the concept that decreased BAT activity, estimated by lower glucose uptake using ^{18}F-FDG PET, is probably not a sign of less thermogenesis but might imply higher insulin resistance, which suggests that glucose uptake is not a reliable method to prove higher BAT-related thermogenesis [23].

2.4 Pitfalls and bias when studying non-shivering thermogenesis in murine models

It is worth noting that most studies in mice are conducted at room temperature (20–23°C), overlooking the fact that the thermoneutral zone of mice and rats is significantly higher (around 30°C). This aspect creates a significant bias because mice are typically housed at room temperature, below their thermoneutral zone, triggering cold adaptations and hyperactivation of the murine BAT [24]. Mild cold in experimental murine models also triggers an increase in food intake to compensate for the heat loss, providing another source of bias. Furthermore, our modern lifestyle involves comfortable temperatures both indoors and outdoors through the use of clothing, heating and insulation, resulting in humans spending most of their lives within their thermoneutral zone (20–22°C). This environmental difference contributes to conflicting data found in the literature about the potential effects of BAT activation and WAT browning in metabolic diseases, particularly when comparing humans and mice [25].

3. Crosstalk between the skeletal muscle and thermogenic adipose tissue

Skeletal muscles play another key role in the prevention of metabolic diseases. Regular physical activity, especially skeletal muscle training and adaptation, promotes glucose uptake by muscle cells and improves insulin sensitivity. This regulates blood sugar levels and reduces the risk of developing type-2 diabetes. Moreover, previous research suggests that browning of the so-called fibro-adipogenic progenitors (FAPs) in muscle can facilitate muscle regeneration by reversing fatty infiltration after injury [26–29]. Although the importance of skeletal muscle in the prevention of metabolic and age-related diseases is recognized, the precise communication between skeletal muscle and brown and beige adipose tissues is not yet fully understood. Particularly through exercise, a complex interaction is postulated to take place between these tissues [30]. However, the intricate mechanisms underlying this crosstalk continue to be researched. These interactions are of particular interest as they could represent potential approaches for the development of new therapies to improve energy expenditure and prevent metabolic diseases more effectively.

4. Batokines and their role in health and disease

Batokines are bioactive molecules secreted by BAT. These signaling factors, which include proteins, peptides, lipids and other bioactive compounds, play a critical role in regulating metabolic homeostasis and inter-organ communication. While the primary function of BAT is thermogenesis—generating heat through the action of uncoupling protein 1 (UCP1) in the mitochondria—research over the past two decades has revealed its additional role as an endocrine organ [31].

Several batokines have been identified, each with distinct roles in promoting metabolic health. For instance, fibroblast growth factor 21 (FGF21) is secreted by BAT during thermogenic activation and acts on peripheral tissues such as the liver and muscles to enhance glucose uptake and lipid oxidation, thereby improving insulin sensitivity and offering protection against obesity. Similarly, interleukin-6 (IL-6) released by BAT contributes to increased energy expenditure and enhanced lipid metabolism while also improving glucose tolerance, distinguishing it from the pro-inflammatory IL-6 secreted by other tissues [32].

Another important batokine is myostatin, a regulator of muscle growth and energy expenditure. Although traditionally associated with skeletal muscle, myostatin secreted by BAT negatively impacts metabolic health, and its inhibition has been shown to boost thermogenesis and systemic energy expenditure [33].

Lipid-based batokines also play a critical role. For example, 12,13-diHOME, a lipid metabolite released during cold exposure, facilitates fatty acid uptake and utilization in skeletal muscle and brown adipocytes, improving metabolic flexibility during heightened energy demand [34]. Similarly, 12-HEPE, derived from omega-3 fatty acids, enhances glucose uptake in peripheral tissues, reduces circulating glucose levels and provides anti-inflammatory effects, making it particularly beneficial in preventing insulin resistance [35].

Together, these diverse batokines illustrate the multifaceted influence of BAT on systemic metabolic health and highlight its potential as a therapeutic target for metabolic disorders.

In conclusion, batokines represent a frontier in metabolic research, offering insights into the endocrine functions of BAT and its systemic impacts on health. By bridging thermogenic activity with inter-organ communication, batokines influence a wide spectrum of physiological processes, from energy balance to immune modulation. Harnessing the therapeutic potential of these molecules could be a potential for the management of metabolic diseases, paving the way for novel treatments targeting obesity, diabetes and cardiovascular disorders.

5. Molecular mechanisms driving BAT activation and WAT browning

The process of converting white fat into brown-like fat, known as "browning" or "beiging," holds significant potential for enhancing metabolic health. Browning can be induced by various stimuli, including cold exposure, beta-adrenergic agonists, specific dietary components, exercise and genetic factors. Beige fat cells, like brown adipocytes, express uncoupling protein 1 (UCP1) and have the capacity to burn calories and produce heat.

Despite the fact that UCP1 is the main protein involved in non-shivering thermogenesis in the BAT [36], studies using UCP1 KO mice have shown unexpectedly adaptation to cold [37], suggesting that there must be UCP1-independent mechanisms able to compensate for the lack of UCP1 to maintain core body temperature under cold-stimulated challenges. Among the known UCP1-independent non-shivering thermogenesis include the futile Ca^{++} cycle [38, 39], the futile lipid [40] and futile creatine [41].

Since subcutaneous adipose tissue has the ability to become "brown" depending on external stimuli, browning of white adipose tissue as well as activation of inactive BAT have been proposed as promising therapeutic approaches against age-related and metabolic diseases [42]. Here, we present some of the most known activators of BAT and WAT browning:

5.1 Cold exposure

Cold exposure is the gold standard mechanism triggering non-shivering thermogenesis. When the body is exposed to cold temperatures, the sympathetic nervous system is activated, releasing norepinephrine (NE). This neurotransmitter binds to beta-adrenergic receptors on brown fat cells, triggering increased levels of intracellular cAMP, which initiates a cascade of events, including transcriptional activation of the cAMP response element-binding protein (CREB), which leads to the activation of UCP1 at the 5′-UTR of the gene and consequently ATP uncoupled thermogenesis [43]. Regular exposure to cold environments, such as through cold showers, ice baths or spending time in cold weather, can increase the amount and activity of brown fat, promoting greater energy expenditure [44–46].

5.2 Thyroid hormone receptors

Thyroid hormones are known as key regulators of energy homeostasis. Mice knockout for all hormone biding nuclear thyroid hormone receptors (TRs) in murine models showed decreased BMR and a slight reduction in body temperature (0.5–1°C lower) compared to the wild-type animals. Of note, exogenous NE treatment failed to activate thermogenesis in these mice under cold acclimation at 4°C. However, decreased thermogenesis was not at the expense of lower UCP1 levels or activity in BAT, but due to less sensitivity to β3-adrenergic stimulation and hence less downstream generation of cAMP, a desensitization that can be restored with higher doses of NE [47].

5.3 Pharmacological treatments

Nowadays, the use of β-2 and β-3 adrenergic receptor (AR) agonists is one of the most studied pharmacological drugs to increase energy expenditure in both rodents and humans. However, many are the concerned due to their undesirable side effects, including a higher prevalence of atherosclerosis and hypertension [48, 49].

Since the discovery of the anti-diabetic effects of β3-AR agonists in murine models in the 1980s, many researchers have become aware of the pharmacological potential that β3-AR agonists may have against metabolic diseases. For example, the β3-AR agonist mirabegron has been suggested to be one of the most promising therapeutic approaches [50, 51]. Approved by the U.S. Food and Drug Administration in 2012, it is known to induce energy expenditure and WAT beiging while presenting low cardiovascular risks at 100 mg dose [52].

However, it was lately known by Blondin et al. that BAT activation in humans, in contrast to mice, is primarily driven by β-2 and not β-3 adrenergic receptors. This might explain the failed attempt to use mirabegron in clinical trials to induce human BAT thermogenesis at the normally prescribed dose [53].

Mechanistic differences between humans and mice, unspecificity of the drugs co-stimulating beta-1 and beta-2 adrenergic receptors and their respective undesired side effects, such as tachycardia and tremors, led to some disappointment in human clinical trials [54]. Of note, administration of the thermogenic drugs such as 2,4-Dinitrophenol (DNP), also used as a pesticide and explosive, may cause hyperthermia, rigidity and high-risk of death due to cardiovascular collapse in case of overdose. Hence, the urge to find safer pharmacological alternatives to increase energy expenditure that can be implemented clinically.

Some of the most clinically promising BAT activator substitutes comprise the use of purine receptor agonists. Gnad et al. showed that adenosine A2A receptor agonist not only enhances energy expenditure and promotes BAT activation and WAT browning, protecting mice from diet-induced obesity but interestingly also counteracts the loss of muscle mass and function during sarcopenia in aged mice [55, 56].

5.4 Melatonin

Melatonin hormone has been shown to regulate energy metabolism affecting BAT activation and volume in a clinical trial in humans. Oral administration of melatonin in patients with melatonin deficiency due to surgical extraction of the pituitary gland of radiotherapy increased BAT volume and improved total blood levels of cholesterol and triglycerides [57].

5.5 Exercise

An exciting aspect to investigate is the potential role of exercise in thermogenesis. Many studies have suggested physical activity as a promising mechanism to counteract the "whitening" effects of aging in brown and beige adipose tissue [58, 59].

One of the mechanisms by which exercise may contribute to thermogenesis is the interaction between skeletal muscle and adipose tissue, which can be mediated by the release of extracellular vesicles (EVs) into the bloodstream [60]. EVs are nanoparticles found in tissues and body fluids and are secreted by cells in response to stress factors such as physical activity and exposure to cold. They play a crucial role in the communication between cells and tissues. Interestingly, some studies in mouse models suggest that exercise stimulates the release of EVs containing microRNAs that regulate the conversion of white-to-beige adipose tissue [61]. However, there are also many studies that provide conflicting data, particularly between humans and mice, probably due to factors such as the temperature in which the mice are housed [62].

If exercise induces browning is still discussed. However, there are several indications that exercise has a browning effect. One of the mechanisms is that physical activity increases the levels of irisin, a hormone released by muscles during exercise. Irisin promotes the browning of white fat and enhances the thermogenic capacity of brown fat [63, 64]. Yet, despite the unquestionable contribution of regular exercise to overall fitness and prevention of weight gain, it is still under investigation whether it could also contribute to the recruitment and activation of brown fat in humans.

5.6 Foods and nutrients

Certain foods and nutrients have been identified as potential activators of brown fat. Capsaicin, the compound responsible for the heat in chili peppers, has been shown to stimulate brown fat activity via the activation of Transient-receptor potential vanilloid 1 (TRPV1) [65]. Similarly, resveratrol, a naturally occurring compound found in red wine, and curcumin, the active component in turmeric, have been found to promote the browning of white fat, converting it into a more metabolically active form that resembles brown fat [66, 67]. Omega-3 fatty acids [68], found in fish oil, have also been linked to increased brown fat activity. Regarding the promising effects of all the mentioned components, the high-dose concentrations used in murine or in vitro studies and the lack of research in human subjects and make it nowadays translationally challenging.

5.7 MicroRNAs

MicroRNAs (miRNAs) are small, non-coding ribonucleic acid (RNA) molecules that play a crucial role in regulating gene expression. Recent research has identified several miRNAs that influence the development and function of brown fat. For instance, miR-196a or inhibition of miR-27b has been shown to promote the browning of white fat [69, 70]. miR-155 is another microRNA that is particularly enriched in brown preadipocytes and whose inhibition enhances brown adipogenesis and browning in white adipocytes and circulatory exosomal-derived miR-92a has been proposed as a biomarker of active BAT in humans [71, 72]. Currently, no miRNAs are known to be used in clinical trials to induce browning in humans. However, understanding the regulatory networks of miRNAs offers new opportunities for traditional therapeutics for the regulation of brown fat activity against metabolic disorders.

6. Therapeutic potential

Harnessing the browning process presents a promising therapeutic strategy for obesity and related metabolic diseases. By increasing the proportion of metabolically active fat, it is possible to enhance overall energy expenditure and reduce adiposity. Therapies aimed at activating brown and beige fat could complement existing weight loss strategies, providing a multifaceted approach to combating obesity, however, further studies are needed.

7. Conclusion

While the potential of brown fat and browning is well-recognized, more research is needed to fully understand the underlying mechanisms and optimize therapeutic approaches. Future studies should focus on identifying novel activators of brown fat, elucidating the role of genetic and epigenetic factors in browning, and developing safe and effective interventions for clinical use without the previously mentioned side effects. Additionally, exploring the interplay between brown fat and other metabolic tissues will provide a more comprehensive understanding of its role in energy homeostasis.

Acknowledgements

The authors would like to thank the Deutsche Forschungsgemeinschaft (DFG, German Research Foundation)—TRR333/1—project# 450149205 Transregio collaborative research center BATenergy.

Conflict of interest

The authors declare no conflict of interest.

Author details

Dominik Tischer and Ana Soriano-Arroquia*
Institute for Pharmacology and Toxicology, Biomedical Center, University of Bonn, Bonn, Germany

*Address all correspondence to: soriano@uni-bonn.de

IntechOpen

© 2025 The Author(s). Licensee IntechOpen. This chapter is distributed under the terms of the Creative Commons Attribution License (http://creativecommons.org/licenses/by/3.0), which permits unrestricted use, distribution, and reproduction in any medium, provided the original work is properly cited.

References

[1] Cinti S. Obesity, Type 2 Diabetes and the Adipose Organ. 2nd ed. Switzerland: Springer International Publishing; 2018. DOI: 10.1007/978-3-319-40522-3. ISBN 978-3-319-40520-9. ISBN 978-3-319-40522-3 (eBook)

[2] Ikeda K, Maretich P, Kajimura S. The common and distinct features of brown and beige adipocytes. Trends in Endocrinology and Metabolism. 2018;**29**:191-200

[3] Virtue S, Vidal-Puig A. Assessment of brown adipose tissue function. Frontiers in Physiology. 2013;**4**:128

[4] Wang QA, Tao C, Gupta RK, Scherer PE. Tracking adipogenesis during white adipose tissue development, expansion and regeneration. Nature Medicine. 2013;**19**:1338-1344

[5] Timmons JA, Wennmalm K, Larsson O, Walden TB, Lassmann T, Petrovic N, et al. Myogenic gene expression signature establishes that brown and white adipocytes originate from distinct cell lineages. Proceedings of the National Academy of Sciences of the United States of America. 2007;**104**:4401-4406

[6] Seale P, Kajimura S, Yang W, Chin S, Rohas LM, Uldry M, et al. Transcriptional control of brown fat determination by PRDM16. Cell Metabolism. 2007;**6**:38-54

[7] Hu E, Tontonoz P, Spiegelman BM. Transdifferentiation of myoblasts by the adipogenic transcription factors PPAR gamma and C/EBP alpha. Proceedings of the National Academy of Sciences of the United States of America. 1995;**92**:9856-9860

[8] Lean MEJ, James WPT, Jennings G, Trayhurn P. Brown adipose tissue uncoupling protein content in human infants, children and adults. Clinical Science. 1986;**71**:291-297

[9] Nedergaard J, Bengtsson T, Cannon B. Unexpected evidence for active brown adipose tissue in adult humans. American Journal of Physiology - Endocrinology and Metabolism. 2007;**293**:E444-E452

[10] van Marken Lichtenbelt WD, Vanhommerig JW, Smulders NM, Drossaerts JMAFL, Kemerink GJ, Bouvy ND, et al. Cold-activated brown adipose tissue in healthy men. The New England Journal of Medicine. 2009;**360**:1500-1508

[11] Cypess AM, Lehman S, Williams G, Tal I, Rodman D, Goldfine AB, et al. Identification and importance of brown adipose tissue in adult humans. The New England Journal of Medicine. 2009;**360**:1509-1517

[12] Virtanen KA, Lidell ME, Orava J, Heglind M, Westergren R, Niemi T, et al. Functional brown adipose tissue in healthy adults. The New England Journal of Medicine. 2009;**360**:1518-1525

[13] Becher T, Palanisamy S, Kramer DJ, Eljalby M, Marx SJ, Wibmer AG, et al. Brown adipose tissue is associated with cardiometabolic health. Nature Medicine. 2021;**27**:58-65

[14] Sellayah D, Sikder D. Orexin restores aging-related brown adipose tissue dysfunction in male mice. Endocrinology. 2014;**155**:485-501

[15] Félix-Soriano E, Sáinz N, Gil-Iturbe E, Collantes M, Fernández-Galilea M, Castilla-Madrigal R, et al. Changes in brown adipose tissue lipid mediator signatures with aging, obesity and DHA

supplementation in female mice. The FASEB Journal. 2021;**35**:e21592

[16] Gohlke S, Zagoriy V, Cuadros Inostroza A, Méret M, Mancini C, Japtok L, et al. Identification of functional lipid metabolism biomarkers of brown adipose tissue aging. Molecular Metabolism. 2019;**24**:1-17

[17] Cao Q, Hersl J, La H, Smith M, Jenkins J, Goloubeva O, et al. A pilot study of FDG PET/CT detects a link between brown adipose tissue and breast cancer. BMC Cancer. 2014;**14**:126

[18] Seki T, Yang Y, Sun X, Lim S, Xie S, Guo Z, et al. Brown-fat-mediated tumour suppression by cold-altered global metabolism. Nature. 2022;**608**:421-428

[19] Levy SB, Leonard WR. The evolutionary significance of human brown adipose tissue: Integrating the timescales of adaptation. Evolutionary Anthropology: Issues, News, and Reviews. 2022;**31**:75-91

[20] Cannon B, Nedergaard J. Nonshivering thermogenesis and its adequate measurement in metabolic studies. The Journal of Experimental Biology. 2011;**214**:242-253

[21] Foster DO, Frydman ML. Nonshivering thermogenesis in the rat. II. Measurements of blood flow with microspheres point to brown adipose tissue as the dominant site of the calorigenesis induced by noradrenaline. Canadian Journal of Physiology and Pharmacology. 1978;**56**(1):110-122. Available from: https://cdnsciencepub.com/doi/10.1139/y78-015

[22] Hanssen MJW, Hoeks J, Brans B, van der Lans AAJJ, Schaart G, van den Driessche JJ, et al. Short-term cold acclimation improves insulin sensitivity in patients with type 2 diabetes mellitus. Nature Medicine. 2015;**21**:863-865

[23] Carpentier AC, Blondin DP. Is stimulation of browning of human adipose tissue a relevant therapeutic target? Annales d'Endocrinologie. 2024;**85**:184-189

[24] Kalinovich AV, de Jong JMA, Cannon B, Nedergaard J. UCP1 in adipose tissues: Two steps to full browning. Biochimie. 2017;**134**:127-137

[25] Zhu Y, Qi Z, Ding S. Exercise-induced adipose tissue thermogenesis and browning: How to explain the conflicting findings? International Journal of Molecular Sciences. 2022;**23**:13142

[26] Lee C, Liu M, Agha O, Kim HT, Feeley BT, Liu X. Beige FAPs transplantation improves muscle quality and shoulder function after massive rotator cuff tears. Journal of Orthopaedic Research. 2020;**38**:1159-1166

[27] Chen S, Bastarrachea RA, Shen J-S, Laviada-Nagel A, Rodriguez-Ayala E, Nava-Gonzalez EJ, et al. Ectopic BAT mUCP-1 overexpression in SKM by delivering a BMP7/PRDM16/PGC-1a gene cocktail or single PRMD16 using non-viral UTMD gene therapy. Gene Therapy. 2018;**25**:497-509

[28] Wang Z, Liu X, Jiang K, Kim H, Kajimura S, Feeley BT. Intramuscular brown fat activation decreases muscle atrophy and fatty infiltration and improves gait after delayed rotator cuff repair in mice. The American Journal of Sports Medicine. 2020;**48**:1590-1600

[29] Davies MR, Garcia S, Liu M, Chi H, Kim HT, Raffai RL, et al. Muscle-derived beige adipose precursors secrete promyogenic exosomes that treat rotator cuff muscle degeneration in mice and are identified in humans by single-cell RNA sequencing. The American Journal of Sports Medicine. 2022;**50**:2247-2257

[30] Sanchez-Delgado G, Martinez-Tellez B, Olza J, Aguilera CM, Gil Á, Ruiz JR. Role of exercise in the activation of brown adipose tissue. Annals of Nutrition & Metabolism. 2015;**67**:21-32

[31] Martins FF, Souza-Mello V, Aguila MB, Mandarim-de-Lacerda CA. Brown adipose tissue as an endocrine organ: Updates on the emerging role of batokines. Hormone Molecular Biology and Clinical Investigation. 2023;**44**:219-227

[32] Stanford KI, Middelbeek RJW, Townsend KL, An D, Nygaard EB, Hitchcox KM, et al. Brown adipose tissue regulates glucose homeostasis and insulin sensitivity. The Journal of Clinical Investigation. 2013;**123**:215-223

[33] Shan T, Liang X, Bi P, Kuang S. Myostatin knockout drives browning of white adipose tissue through activating the AMPK-PGC1α-Fndc5 pathway in muscle. The FASEB Journal. 2013;**27**:1981-1989

[34] Stanford KI, Lynes MD, Takahashi H, Baer LA, Arts PJ, May FJ, et al. 12,13-diHOME: An exercise-induced lipokine that increases skeletal muscle fatty acid uptake. Cell Metabolism. 2018;**27**:1111-1120.e3

[35] Leiria LO, Wang C-H, Lynes MD, Yang K, Shamsi F, Sato M, et al. 12-lipoxygenase regulates cold adaptation and glucose metabolism by producing the omega-3 lipid 12-HEPE from brown fat. Cell Metabolism. 2019;**30**:768-783.e7

[36] Nedergaard J, Golozoubova V, Matthias A, Asadi A, Jacobsson A, Cannon B. UCP1: The only protein able to mediate adaptive non-shivering thermogenesis and metabolic inefficiency. Biochimica et Biophysica Acta (BBA) - Bioenergetics. 2001;**1504**:82-106

[37] Meyer CW, Willershäuser M, Jastroch M, Rourke BC, Fromme T, Oelkrug R, et al. Adaptive thermogenesis and thermal conductance in wild-type and UCP1-KO mice. American Journal of Physiology. Regulatory, Integrative and Comparative Physiology. 2010;**299**:R1396-R1406

[38] Ikeda K, Kang Q, Yoneshiro T, Camporez JP, Maki H, Homma M, et al. UCP1-independent signaling involving SERCA2b-mediated calcium cycling regulates beige fat thermogenesis and systemic glucose homeostasis. Nature Medicine. 2017;**23**:1454-1465

[39] Bal NC, Periasamy M. Uncoupling of sarcoendoplasmic reticulum calcium ATPase pump activity by sarcolipin as the basis for muscle non-shivering thermogenesis. Philosophical Transactions of the Royal Society of London. Series B, Biological Sciences. 2020;**375**:20190135

[40] Oeckl J, Janovska P, Adamcova K, Bardova K, Brunner S, Dieckmann S, et al. Loss of UCP1 function augments recruitment of futile lipid cycling for thermogenesis in murine brown fat. Molecular Metabolism. 2022;**61**:101499

[41] Kazak L, Chouchani ET, Jedrychowski MP, Erickson BK, Shinoda K, Cohen P, et al. A creatine-driven substrate cycle enhances energy expenditure and thermogenesis in beige fat. Cell. 2015;**163**:643-655

[42] Barbatelli G, Murano I, Madsen L, Hao Q, Jimenez M, Kristiansen K, et al. The emergence of cold-induced brown adipocytes in mouse white fat depots is determined predominantly by white to brown adipocyte transdifferentiation.

American Journal of Physiology - Endocrinology and Metabolism. 2010;**298**:E1244-E1253

[43] Villarroya F, Peyrou M, Giralt M. Transcriptional regulation of the uncoupling protein-1 gene. Biochimie. 2017;**134**:86-92

[44] Søberg S, Löfgren J, Philipsen FE, Jensen M, Hansen AE, Ahrens E, et al. Altered brown fat thermoregulation and enhanced cold-induced thermogenesis in young, healthy, winter-swimming men. Cell Reports Medicine. 2021;**2**:100408

[45] Gordon K, Blondin DP, Friesen BJ, Tingelstad HC, Kenny GP, Haman F. Seven days of cold acclimation substantially reduces shivering intensity and increases nonshivering thermogenesis in adult humans. Journal of Applied Physiology. 1985;**2019**(126):1598-1606

[46] Blondin DP, Labbé SM, Tingelstad HC, Noll C, Kunach M, Phoenix S, et al. Increased brown adipose tissue oxidative capacity in cold-acclimated humans. The Journal of Clinical Endocrinology and Metabolism. 2014;**99**:E438-E446

[47] Golozoubova V, Gullberg H, Matthias A, Cannon B, Vennström B, Nedergaard J. Depressed thermogenesis but competent brown adipose tissue recruitment in mice devoid of all hormone-binding thyroid hormone receptors. Molecular Endocrinology. 2004;**18**:384-401

[48] Sui W, Li H, Yang Y, Jing X, Xue F, Cheng J, et al. Bladder drug mirabegron exacerbates atherosclerosis through activation of brown fat-mediated lipolysis. Proceedings of the National Academy of Sciences of the United States of America. 2019;**116**:10937-10942

[49] Farzam K, Kidron A, Lakhkar AD. Adrenergic drugs. In: StatPearls. Treasure Island, FL: StatPearls Publishing; 2024. Available from: http://www.ncbi.nlm.nih.gov/books/NBK534230/

[50] Bel JS, Tai TC, Khaper N, Lees SJ. Mirabegron: The most promising adipose tissue beiging agent. Physiological Reports. 2021;**9**:e14779

[51] Cypess AM, Weiner LS, Roberts-Toler C, Elía EF, Kessler SH, Kahn PA, et al. Activation of human brown adipose tissue by a β3-adrenergic receptor agonist. Cell Metabolism. 2015;**21**:33-38

[52] Loh RKC, Formosa MF, La Gerche A, Reutens AT, Kingwell BA, Carey AL. Acute metabolic and cardiovascular effects of mirabegron in healthy individuals. Diabetes, Obesity and Metabolism. 2019;**21**:276-284

[53] Blondin DP, Nielsen S, Kuipers EN, Severinsen MC, Jensen VH, Miard S, et al. Human brown adipocyte thermogenesis is driven by β2-AR stimulation. Cell Metabolism. 2020;**32**:287-300.e7

[54] de Souza CJ, Burkey BF. Beta3-adrenoceptor agonists as anti-diabetic and anti-obesity drugs in humans. Current Pharmaceutical Design;**7**:1433-1449

[55] Gnad T, Scheibler S, von Kügelgen I, Scheele C, Kilić A, Glöde A, et al. Adenosine activates brown adipose tissue and recruits beige adipocytes via A2A receptors. Nature. 2014;**516**:395-399

[56] Gnad T, Navarro G, Lahesmaa M, Reverte-Salisa L, Copperi F, Cordomi A, et al. Adenosine/A2B receptor signaling ameliorates the effects of aging and counteracts obesity. Cell Metabolism. 2020;**32**:56-70.e7

[57] Halpern B, Mancini MC, Bueno C, Barcelos IP, de Melo ME, Lima MS, et al. Melatonin increases brown adipose tissue volume and activity in patients with

melatonin deficiency: A proof-of-concept study. Diabetes. 2019;**68**:947-952

[58] Nirengi S, Stanford K. Brown adipose tissue and aging: A potential role for exercise. Experimental Gerontology. 2023;**178**:112218

[59] Nigro P, Vamvini M, Yang J, Caputo T, Ho L-L, Carbone NP, et al. Exercise training remodels inguinal white adipose tissue through adaptations in innervation, vascularization, and the extracellular matrix. Cell Reports. 2023;**42**(4):112392. Available from: https://www.cell.com/cell-reports/abstract/S2211-1247(23)00403-5

[60] Rome S. Muscle and adipose tissue communicate with extracellular vesicles. International Journal of Molecular Sciences. 2022;**23**:7052

[61] Di W, Amdanee N, Zhang W, Zhou Y. Long-term exercise-secreted extracellular vesicles promote browning of white adipocytes by suppressing miR-191a-5p. Life Sciences. 2020;**263**:118464

[62] McKie GL, Wright DC. The confounding effects of sub-thermoneutral housing temperatures on aerobic exercise-induced adaptations in mouse subcutaneous white adipose tissue. Biology Letters. 2021;**17**:20210171

[63] Shi H, Hao X, Sun Y, Zhao Y, Wang Y, Cao X, et al. Exercise-inducible circulating extracellular vesicle irisin promotes browning and the thermogenic program in white adipose tissue. Acta Physiologica. 2024;**240**:e14103

[64] Islam MR, Valaris S, Young MF, Haley EB, Luo R, Bond SF, et al. Exercise hormone irisin is a critical regulator of cognitive function. Nature Metabolism. 2021;**3**:1058-1070

[65] Baskaran P, Nazminia K, Frantz J, O'Neal J, Thyagarajan B. Mice lacking endogenous TRPV1 express reduced levels of thermogenic proteins and are susceptible to diet-induced obesity and metabolic dysfunction. FEBS Letters. 2021;**595**:1768-1781

[66] Wang S, Liang X, Yang Q, Fu X, Rogers CJ, Zhu M, et al. Resveratrol induces brown-like adipocyte formation in white fat through activation of AMP-activated protein kinase (AMPK) α1. International Journal of Obesity. 2015;**39**:967-976

[67] Lone J, Choi JH, Kim SW, Yun JW. Curcumin induces brown fat-like phenotype in 3T3-L1 and primary white adipocytes. Journal of Nutritional Biochemistry. 2016;**27**:193-202

[68] Kim M, Goto T, Yu R, Uchida K, Tominaga M, Kano Y, et al. Fish oil intake induces UCP1 upregulation in brown and white adipose tissue via the sympathetic nervous system. Scientific Reports. 2015;**5**:18013

[69] Mori M, Nakagami H, Rodriguez-Araujo G, Nimura K, Kaneda Y. Essential role for miR-196a in brown adipogenesis of white fat progenitor cells. PLoS Biology. 2012;**10**:e1001314

[70] Tang Y, Yang L-J, Liu H, Song Y-J, Yang Q-Q, Liu Y, et al. Exosomal miR-27b-3p secreted by visceral adipocytes contributes to endothelial inflammation and atherogenesis. Cell Reports. 2023;**42**:111948

[71] Chen Y, Siegel F, Kipschull S, Haas B, Fröhlich H, Meister G, et al. miR-155 regulates differentiation of brown and beige adipocytes via a bistable circuit. Nature Communications. 2013;**4**:1769

[72] Chen Y, Buyel JJ, Hanssen MJW, Siegel F, Pan R, Naumann J, et al. Exosomal microRNA miR-92a concentration in serum reflects human brown fat activity. Nature Communications. 2016;**7**:11420

Chapter 6

In Vitro Differentiation of Beige/Brown Adipocytes for the Treatment of Metabolic Diseases

Amine Bouchekioua, Olivier Pourquié and Alicia Mayeuf-Louchart

Abstract

Brown adipose tissue is responsible for non-shivering thermogenesis, controlling temperature regulation in newborns and childhood, and then in adults under cold conditions. However, its physiological functions are broader and include endocrine functions, regulation of glucose homeostasis and insulin sensitivity, as well as triglyceride clearance. BAT activity is inversely correlated with body mass index (BMI), and cold-induced thermogenesis is significantly lower in people with excess weight and obesity. Therefore, brown adipocyte transplantation represents a new perspective for the treatment of diabetes, obesity and their cardiovascular and metabolic consequences. Several strategies have been designed to obtain brown adipocytes *in vitro*, notably based on the differentiation of human pluripotent stem cells (PSCs). In this chapter, we review the latest findings on the embryonic development of the different adipocyte lineages, which have laid the foundations for PSCs differentiation protocols. We discuss the most recent technologies and their limitations, and the pharmacological approaches to stimulate brown adipocyte activity *in vivo*.

Keywords: brown adipocytes, PSCs, cell therapy, beiging, cell differentiation

1. Introduction

Diabetes and obesity are widespread disorders in modern societies, and their cardiovascular, hormonal, and metabolic consequences have a significant and growing impact on public health [1–3]. Currently, the treatment of diabetes is daily, laborious and intrusive. Moreover, although there are several behavioral, hormonal, or surgical treatments for obesity, they sometimes have significant side effects and are not always effective for every patient [4].

Several studies have been conducted in recent years to find new treatments to these disorders. Among them, targeting brown adipose tissue (BAT) has been proposed as a potential strategy. Initially identified in newborns for its heat production and thermoregulatory properties, it has been shown that BAT is also present in adults in small deposits. In addition to its role in thermoregulation, BAT has endocrine functions [5, 6], allows triglyceride clearance [7], and regulates glucose homeostasis and insulin sensitivity [8]. Brown adipocytes express the mitochondrial protein UCP1 (Uncoupled protein 1), which uncouples the respiratory chain from ATP synthase, releasing energy in the form of heat instead of ATP (Adenosine triphosphate) [9]. Some white adipocytes can also be converted to thermogenic cells called beige adipocytes, which share similar properties to brown adipocytes upon exposure to cold or drug treatments such as Forskolin [10]. This illustrates the adaptability of adipose tissues to environmental conditions. Another similar example is the transdifferentiation of white adipocytes into "pink" adipocytes in the mammary gland during pregnancy [11].

Transplantation of healthy BAT tissues into mice improves glycemia and insulin sensitivity in type 1 (T1D) [12, 13] and type 2 (T2D) [14] diabetic non-obese animals. This confirms the high potential of BAT for cell therapy approaches to treat these diseases. Research has also been carried out to pharmacologically activate the beiging of white adipose tissue (WAT), but with no real success so far [15]. Another new strategy currently being explored is to generate thermogenic adipose tissue *in vitro* for transplantation. With the emergence of personal medicine and regenerative therapies, efforts are also deployed to generate brown adipocytes *in vitro* from human pluripotent stem cells (PSCs). PSCs are of interest for regenerative medicine because they can be generated from the patient's own cells, allowing both autologous engraftment and infinite production of cells.

In this chapter, we will focus first on reviewing the lineages and roles of heat-producing adipocytes, and the importance of these cells for human metabolism and health. Then, we summarize the strategies developed to pharmacologically stimulate adipocyte beiging and discuss the latest advances in obtaining brown/beige adipocytes *in vitro* for transplantation.

2. Functions and origins of adipocytes involved in non-shivering thermogenesis

2.1 Discovery and functions of BAT

Human brown fat was identified as a tissue involved in non-shivering thermogenesis in newborns. It allows thermoregulation during the early stages of life, when heat production by muscle shivering is not yet possible [16]. Its total regression in adulthood, initially presumed, was refuted thanks to imaging approaches [17] combining Positron emission tomography (PET) and computer tomography (CT) with a fluorodeoxyglucose tracer (18F-FDG) [18]. This uncovered region of high glucose uptake, subsequently identified as BAT.

Brown adipocytes are characterized by expression of UCP1, a transmembrane protein located in the inner mitochondrial membrane. UCP1 enables heat production allowing dissipation of the proton gradient created by the mitochondrial respiratory chain. UCP1 allows the dissipation of energy as heat instead of storing it as ATP. Brown adipocytes exhibit multilocular lipid droplets, with each droplet composed of triglycerides. During embryonic development, lipid droplets are formed within glycogen clusters, which are progressively degraded [19]. Lipid droplets are closely associated with glycogen granules, improving substrate utilization and increasing heat generation efficiency. This thermogenic system uses ß-Oxidation and the Krebs cycle to respectively burn fatty acids and glucose as fuel in the mitochondria. This explains the brown fat ability to increase triglyceride [7] and glucose [8] clearance.

2.2 Role of BAT in metabolic disorders

Obesity is associated with hyperplasic and hypertrophic white adipocytes that release free fatty acids, pro-inflammatory factors and reactive oxygen species (ROS). As a result, inflammation and lipotoxicity affect several tissues, such as muscles, liver or BAT. These defects, which also lead to organelle dysfunction, are the main cause of insulin resistance [20]. The inflammatory process involves TNF-α [21], which is a pro-inflammatory factor promoting the activity of several factors directly targeting insulin receptors on their serine residues [20, 22].

A number of studies have highlighted the close link between BAT activity and metabolic disorders [23]. Among them, Becher et al. recently studied the correlation between BAT and pathophysiological phenotypes [3]. This retrospective case-control study of patients diagnosed with cancer, monitored BAT activity using 18F-FDG PET-CT. Imaging was used to classify patients into two categories, BAT-positive (BAT+) and BAT-negative (BAT-). Results showed a positive correlation between BAT activity and lower body mass index (BMI), younger age and exposure to lower temperatures. Data collected during cold seasons showed significantly higher BAT activity. The incidence of various cardiovascular and metabolic diseases was assessed in the BAT+ and BAT- populations. Patients with obesity identified as BAT+ had a lower risk of developing complications than BAT- with a similar BMI, showing a protective effect of BAT against dyslipidemia, type 2 diabetes (T2D), cardiovascular and cerebrovascular afflictions. This analysis showed better glycemic regulation, lower blood triglyceride levels and higher levels of high-density lipoprotein (HDL) in the BAT+ group.

To conclude, brown fat presence is associated with better cardiometabolic health. Its activity is higher in women, young people, in a context of non-obesity and at cold temperatures [3].

2.3 The four different adipocyte types and their lineages

Adipocytes are classified into four categories based on color: white, brown, beige and pink. White adipocytes are the most commonly known adipocytes, involved in lipid storage and characterized by a single lipid droplet occupying the majority of the cytoplasm. Brown but also beige (or brite) adipocytes are cells involved in non-shivering thermogenesis [24, 25]. Beige adipocytes are white adipocytes which have the capacity to express UCP1 when stimulated. After stimulation by exposure to cold [26] or with activation of the Peroxisome Proliferator-activated Receptor γ (PPARγ) [24], UCP1 begins to be expressed in these cells, which then start to adopt a phenotype resembling brown adipocytes [27]. However, beige adipocytes are not just an inducible version of brown adipocytes, as they exhibit different cell markers, anatomical location, and they have a different embryologic origin [28].

Another type of adipocyte discovered recently are the pink adipocytes, only present during pregnancy, lactation and post-lactation. They arise from the transdifferentiation of subcutaneous white adipocytes into milk-producing glands [11]. Pink adipocytes are named for their lipid-rich composition. They are parenchymatous adipose organ cells containing large cytoplasmic lipid droplets whose function is to produce milk. Characteristics, roles and localization of each cell type is summarized in the **Figure 1A**.

To better understand adipocyte plasticity, with transdifferentiation and phenotypic changes, it is important to look at the developmental origin of these cell types

(**Figure 1B**). After gastrulation, mammalian embryos are composed of three cell layers: endoderm, mesoderm and ectoderm. The embryonic mesoderm is divided in three main regions: the lateral plate mesoderm, which gives rise to most of the WAT;

A

Adipocyte	UCP1	Mitochondria	Location in human	Main role
Brown	High expression	High density	Supraclavicular Paravertebral Perivasicular Periviscus Interscapurlar	Thermogenesis Energy expenditure Triglycerides clearance Regulation of glucose homeostasis Regulation of insulin sensitivity Endocrine
White	None	Low density	Visceral Subcutaneous Epididymal	Energy storage Endocrine
Beige	Medium expression	Medium density	Supraclavicular Subcutaneous	Thermogenesis Energy expenditure Triglycerides clearance Regulation of glucose homeostasis Regulation of insulin sensitivity Endocrine
Pink	None	Low density	Mammary gland	Milk production during pregnancy, lactation and post-lactation periods

B

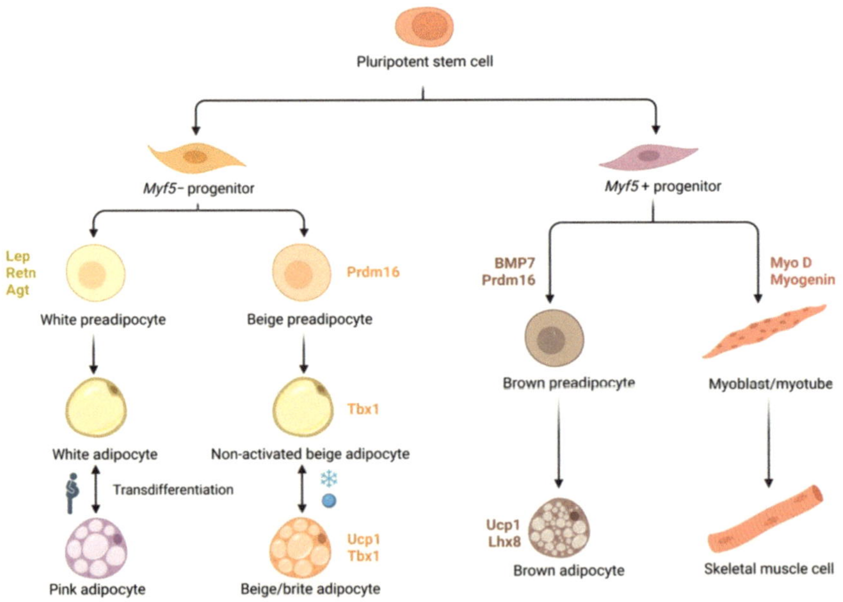

Figure 1.
Origins and description of the four different types of adipocytes. (A) Table summarizing the characteristics and localization of each human adipose tissue. (B) Diagram showing the different adipose lineages derived from pluripotent stem cells during the physiological development in mouse. Myf5-negative (Myf5-) progenitors give rise to white, beige and pink precursors, while Myf5-positive (Myf5+) lead to brown adipocytes and skeletal muscle cells. Beige and white adipocytes share the same phenotype at a basal state, but beige adipocytes can adopt a brown-like phenotype after exposure to low temperatures or drug treatment such as Forskolin. Leptin (Lep), Resistin (Retn) and Angiotensinogen (Agt) are differentially expressed between white and beige preadipocytes. Pink adipocytes result from white transdifferentiation during pregnancy and lactation.

the intermediate mesoderm, which gives rise to kidneys and gonads; and the paraxial mesoderm, which contains the presomitic mesoderm (PSM). The PSM undergoes a mesenchymal-epithelial transition that results in the formation of somites. Brown adipocyte progenitors originate from the dorsal part of the somite, the dermomyotome. They share a common progenitor (MYF5+, PAX7+) with skeletal muscles and dermis (**Figure 1B**) [10].

We performed a single cell RNA sequencing analysis [29] of the dorsal tissue of developing mouse embryos and identified a cluster, at E11.5, containing fibroblastic progenitors of bone, cartilage, smooth muscles, connective tissues, dermis and brown adipocytes which express *Pdgfr-α* and *Hic1*. Bioinformatics analyzes suggest that these progenitors give rise to brown adipocyte precursors which express *Ebf2* and *Pparγ*. These precursors give rise to a population of embryonic brown adipocytes expressing *Ucp1* and *Cidea* which is first detected at E15.5 [29, 30]. Our work also identified *Gata6* as a selective marker transiently expressed in the brown adipocyte lineage.

Beige and white precursors develop from different MYF5-negative cell lineages, like neural crest [31] or lateral mesoderm [32]. Like brown adipocytes, beige adipocytes express *Prmd16* during their differentiation [33]. Pink adipocytes arise from white adipocytes during lactation episodes by transdifferentiation [11]. During pregnancy, subcutaneous white adipocytes undergo structural remodeling resulting in enlarged endoplasmic reticulum and Golgi apparatus and splitting of the large lipid droplets into numerous small units [34]. At the end of the lactation episode, pink adipocytes re-adopt a white phenotype.

Understanding the development of these tissues is of particular interest for establishing strategies based on the production of differentiated brown adipocytes *in vitro* in a therapeutic perspective against metabolic disorders.

3. Pharmacological strategies to stimulate the activity of brown adipocytes

Pharmacological approaches aimed at stimulating brown adipocytes activity or at inducing the browning/beiging [35, 36] of white adipocytes have been tested as potential strategies to improve metabolic disorders. Increasing differentiation, proliferation and activation of brown/beige adipocytes has been shown to promote energy expenditure, insulin sensitivity and anti-inflammatory processes in animal models [37].

One example is the modulation of the RAR-related orphan receptor alpha (RORα) *in vivo* with an inverse-agonist (SR3335), which results in an increased UCP1 expression in BAT and WAT of wild-type mice [35]. RORα-deficient mice show a beiging phenotype with increased UCP1 expression and a higher metabolic rate [38, 39]. Antagonizing RORα with SR3335 *in vivo* successfully resulted in beiging the WAT and improving metabolism of mice with diet-induced obesity [35]. However, as RORα is an ubiquitous nuclear factor, any inhibition treatment would most likely result in a wide range of side effects.

Another approach is based on a serotonin reuptake inhibitor, the Fluoxetine, which can increase mitochondrial biogenesis and activation in different tissues [40]. In a population of young and obese rats, chronic Fluoxetine treatment was shown to induce beiging [40]. However, this also results in an increase in oxidative stress [40], meaning that this strategy would not be suitable for patients with diabetes. Serotonin reuptake inhibitors are mainly used to treat depression and anxiety troubles and their side effects, like somnolence, headaches, and tremors are well-known.

The second pharmacological axis is the *in vivo* activation of BAT by stimulating its regulators. Four class of drugs have been described to activate BAT [41]: class 1, such as mirabegron [42] consists of β3-adrenergic agonists; class 2 acts on the norepinephrine transporter, thus activating β3-adrenergic receptor; class 3 activates PPARγ; class 4 includes other strategies and natural products. Class 1 and 2 are stimulating the sympathetic nervous system, which activates BAT through the β3-adrenergic pathway. These drug-based strategies showed several limits, such as lack of specificity resulting in psychiatric and cardiac side effects. BAT regulation is complex and involves many different players. In man, in contrast to rodent, brown adipose-driven thermogenesis is not activated by the β3 but by the β2-adrenergic receptor (β2-AR) stimulation [43]. Former strategies relied on high doses of β3-adrenergic agonists, as their thermogenic effect were due to off-targeting β2-AR stimulation [43]. A randomized trial to evaluate the effect of the β2-AR agonist, Salbutamol [44] showed a positive effect on BAT glucose uptake without altering uptake in white adipose and skeletal muscle. However, the trial only included young and healthy men, which is the population with the highest BAT presence [44]. Furthermore, Salbutamol is usually used to treat respiratory diseases, and its effects are not expected to be restricted to BAT. Such a treatment could lead to a wide range of side effects if the drug is not delivered in a tissue specific fashion.

4. New strategies for the generation of beige adipocytes

4.1 Engineering beige adipocytes with CRISPR

Human "brown-like" adipocytes, or HUMBLEs [45], are the result of beiging engineering, using a CRISPR-based Synergistic Activation Mediator (CRISPR-SAM) technology to overexpress UCP1 in white pre-adipocytes in culture (**Figure 2A**). This technique uses a defective Cas9 protein, dCas9, which can bind DNA but is unable to fulfill its endonuclease function [51]. It is fused with transcriptional activators such as VP64, p65 or HSF1, resulting in overexpression of the targeted gene. This system is highly specific thanks to the RNA guides designed to target *UCP1*. Overexpression of UCP1 in HUMBLEs increased intracellular AMP concentrations and phosphorylation of AMPK. This results in higher mitochondrial biogenesis [52] with active UCP1, conferring on HUMBLEs a functional "brown-like" phenotype. These human cells were then transplanted in mice under high fat diet and results show that metabolic parameters such as body weight, energy expenditure, glucose homeostasis, insulin sensitivity and triglyceride clearance were improved over long term (up to 12 weeks) [45]. However, assessment of glucose uptake *in vivo* using a radiotracer showed no difference between transplanted- HUMBLES and control mice. The healthier phenotype of transplanted mice was not due to the autonomous metabolic properties of the engineered cells, but due to the increased activity of endogenous BAT. Transplanted HUMBLEs have been shown to activate the endogenous BAT, through the production of nitric oxide (NO) [45]. NO is known to regulate mitochondrial function, increasing expression of thermogenic genes and leading to the beiging of white adipocytes [53].

In conclusion, these cells are not as efficient as mature brown or beige adipocytes, due to their inability to increase their glucose uptake *in vivo*. However, as they fulfill the remaining functions of beige/brown adipocytes and stimulate endogenous brown fat, they remain a potential target for the treatment of diabetes and obesity.

A

Strategy of generation	Initial cell type	Final cell type
CRISPR-induced overexpression of UCP1 (HUMBLEs)	White preadipocytes from an immortalized line	Bio-engineered beige adipocytes with a brown-like high UCP1 expression
Angiogenesis induction followed by beige induction	Beige preadipocytes from panniculectomy. Adipogenesis stimulates its proliferation	Beige adipocytes inducted with Forskolin

B

Protocol	Initial cell type	Final cell type	Observations
Nishio and al. 2012 Beiging by hematopoietic cocktail exposure	2D human iPSCs and hESCs culture	2D functional beige adipocytes	The protocol does not follow the *in vivo* pathway Short-term efficiency *in vivo* Aiming for brown cultures, but beige transcriptomic signature
Carobbio and al. 2021 Differentiation going through the paraxial mesoderm stage	2D human iPSCs culture	2D embryonic brown adipocytes	The protocol does not follow the *in vivo* pathway : No WNT and BMP modulation High death rates during differentiation and dissociation.
Zhang and al. 2020 Differentiation going through the paraxial mesoderm stage	2D human iPSCs culture	2D embryonic brown adipocytes	High death rates during differentiation and dissociation. The protocol does not follow the *in vivo* pathway : empirical strategy Short-term efficiency *in vivo*
Rao and al. 2022 Differentiation going through the GATA6 precursor stage	2D human iPSCs culture	2D embryonic brown adipocytes	High number of brown adipocytes generated. Culture transcriptionally close to *in vivo* tissues High death rate during dissociation.
Wang and al. 2023 3D differentiation, cells are not attached to the well	3D human brown progenitors cultures (organoids)	Mature BAT organoids	Low death rates during differentiation Grafts active 5 months after transplantation

Figure 2.
Differentiation strategies for non-shivering thermogenic cells. (A) Table comparing the two strategies presented for beige differentiation. The upper strategy is the HUMBLE strategy, achieved by overexpressing UCP1 through CRISPR technology [44]. The second is the discovery of beige adipocytes proliferation upon co-culture with capillaries and exposure to angiogenic factors [46]. (B) Comparative table of the five strategies leading to the differentiation of brown adipocytes [29, 47–50].

4.2 Obtaining beige adipocytes using angiogenic factors

Human adipocyte precursors develop around newly formed vascular networks [54]. Angiogenesis is required for proliferation of adipose tissue during development and is involved in hypertrophic expansion during adulthood [46]. This link between adipogenesis and angiogenesis, has led to the hypothesis that pro-angiogenic factors may be involved in adipocytes differentiation and proliferation. This could be explained by the need for a strong vascular network in the vicinity of adipocytes to enable them to perform their functions, such as glucose and triglyceride uptake, endocrine secretions, etc.

To assess a potential influence of capillaries on adipocytes development, Min et al. [55] developed an *in vitro* system in which adipocytes are co-cultured with microvessels (**Figure 2A**). This protocol uses adipose tissue harvested from individuals who have been subjected to panniculectomy, i.e. the ablation of excessive skin and subcutaneous fat, often practiced after important weight loss. These samples were cultured *in vitro* with angiogenic factors such as VEGF (vascular endothelial growth factor), hEGF (human epidermal growth factor) or hFGF-B (human fibroblast growth factor B). This process results in the formation of capillaries *in vitro* [55]. Each capillary gives rise to sprouts, and the cells located at the tips of these sprouts organizes themselves into thicker structures. These structures are composed of various types of cells, including both endothelial and non-endothelial cells [55, 56]. To assess the presence of adipocytes progenitors in these vessel-like structures, the medium was replaced by an adipogenic cocktail, which induced differentiation into adipocytes [55]. As a result, vessels are surrounded by cells exhibiting multiple lipid droplets, leading to the conclusion that human adipose progenitors' growth is simultaneous with the growth of capillaries. This process was found to be highly reliant on pro-angiogenic growth factors. A question remains: are these white or beige-inducible adipocytes [55]? To find out, adipose tissue taken from the previous culture was exposed to Forskolin, an activator of adenylate cyclase acting as a beiging signal. Results show the presence of beige adipocytes within the culture. Transplantation of these cells into mice fed with high fat-diet shows improved glucose homeostasis. However, triglyceride clearance and changes in body weight were not assessed [55].

5. Differentiating PSCs into thermogenic brown adipocytes

Transplantation of BAT from healthy mice to mice with obesity, type 1 [12, 13] or type 2 [14] diabetes rescues the pathological phenotype. However, this involves the use of healthy tissue taken from an individual and requires finding a way to overcome immune rejection. Moreover, the number of transplants would be limited by the number of donors. Developing a treatment for those epidemic afflictions requires an unlimited source of brown adipocytes for large-scale processing. iPSCs are very interesting in this respect [47]. They represent an unlimited source of cells that can be converted into mature beige/brown adipocytes. They can also be used for autologous treatment, thus circumventing immune reaction. Each patient provides their own cells, which are reprogrammed to the pluripotent state with Yamanaka factors, differentiated *in vitro* into brown adipocytes and then transplanted. Efforts are underway to optimize this strategy, but above all it is crucial to succeed in developing mature brown adipocytes from the renewable source of iPSCs.

5.1 Development of PSCs-derived brown/beige adipocytes

Different protocols had been developed to obtain brown adipocytes from PSCs. Among them, Nishio et al. [48] produced thermogenic adipocytes from PSCs by culturing them with a medium supplemented with vascular endothelial growth factor (VEGF), interleukin-6 (IL6), fms-related tyrosine kinase 3 ligand (FLT3LG) and KIT ligand (KITLG). Subcutaneous injection of their cells in mice successfully reduced levels of glucose and triglycerides after a few hours in a context of fasting or after high fat-diet, but no long-term data were provided. Zhang et al. [57] (**Figure 2B**) studied the markers expressed during the differentiation of adipocytes (**Figure 1B**). Brown adipocytes arise from the paraxial mesoderm, while the white and beige mostly originate from the splanchnic mesoderm [58]. Their study concludes that Nishio et al. [48] and other previous protocols produced beige adipocytes, which need to be induced to express UCP1, and which have a weaker thermogenic function due to their lower concentration of mitochondria.

In an effort to obtain brown adipocytes from iPSCs, we recently developed a new protocol based an analysis of *in vivo* development of brown adipocytes in mice [29]. We analyzed the transcriptomic profile of mouse inter-scapular BAT (iBAT) at different embryological stages [19, 29]. By using single cell RNA-sequencing, we identified of a population of Gata6-positive brown adipocyte precursors appearing at E13.5 (Embryonic day). We also identified signaling molecules and transcription factors exhibiting specific regulation during brown adipocytes differentiation. Based on the protocol of Chal et al. [49, 59] for muscle generation *in vitro*, we conducted differentiation of human iPSCs to paraxial mesoderm, somite identity and PAX7-positive precursors. Based on our *in vivo* findings, we developed a 2D culture protocol to differentiate PAX7-positive cultures first toward GATA6-positive precursors and then into UCP1-positive cells after 40 days of culture. This protocol therefore generates brown adipocyte by following the differentiation pathway recapitulating the normal developmental trajectory of brown adipocytes *in vivo*.

Zhang et al. [57] and Carobbio et al. [60] have also elaborated protocols for generating BAT starting with paraxial mesoderm induction. However, the scarcity of information BAT development prevented them to benchmark the subsequent steps of their protocol against brown adipocyte differentiation *in vivo*. In contrast, in our study, the nature and timing of administration of the different factors used in the protocol was inferred based on the scRNAseq analysis of brown adipocytes development *in vivo*. For instance, a major difference is the use of BMP7 by Zhang et al. [57] at day 8 of culture, when cells are still at the somite/dermomyotome stage. In contrast, we [29] introduce it at day 20, at a stage when PAX7+ brown fat progenitors have been generated. Moreover, these two studies differ on the use of TGF-β. While we suggest that TGF-β promotes adipogenesis at a progenitor stage, Zhang et al. are inhibiting it at this stage. Transcriptomic comparison of BAT generated with these three protocols showed that the tissue obtained with our protocol is closer to human BAT [29].

Zhang et al. [57] performed injections in immunodeficient mice with diabetes to assess the functionality of the cells differentiated with their protocol. They reported a higher body temperature and a significant increase in global metabolism in the injected mice. However, the long-term impact of these grafts has not been investigated.

5.2 Development of 3D BAT organoids for transplantation

Previous strategies were focused on the development of functional brown adipocytes in 2D cultures from PSCs. These techniques yielded non-optimal results in terms of their anti-obesity and anti-diabetic effect in the long-term *in vivo* compared to transplantation of mouse tissue to an obese or diabetic one. The survival rate of adipocytes during cultures, preparation and transplantation are very low, reducing the efficiency of the treatment [50, 61]. Adipocytes are very fragile cells and they do not survive well the dissociation process [50]. Furthermore, Liu et al. [50]

demonstrated that injection of brown adipocytes differentiated *in vitro* from 2D cultures results in the death of 97.3% of them after 1 week.

To increase tissue cohesion and avoid the critical step of enzymatic dissociation of cultures, Wang et al. recently developed a 3D model based on an immortalized brown adipocyte progenitor line (**Figure 2B**) [61]. This enables BAT organoids to be formed, cultured in suspension with their differentiation medium. Centrifugation in non-adherent wells leading to the aggregation of stem cells, forming a small disk. The differentiation process is very similar to the 2D protocols, but the cells form aggregates in suspension, and culture takes place on agitated plates. These organoids were cultured in thermoreversible hydrogels [62], before being injected into the kidneys of mice with obesity and induced type 2 diabetes. This protocol increased triglycerides clearance, insulin sensitivity and glucose uptake, and decreased body mass in obese models. To complete the functional evaluation of their 3D structures, they measured plasma adipokines [61]. The grafts survived for 5 months, expressing UCP1 and fulfilling their thermogenic and metabolic roles. In this study, organoids were not generated from iPSCs, but using progenitors isolated from the resection and purification of a patient's adipose tissue [61].

6. Conclusion

Cell therapy involving BAT transplant is a promising strategy to treat disorders as obesity, diabetes, and their cardio-metabolic consequences. This strategy is competing with pharmaceutical treatments, which aim to activate BAT *in vivo* directly. Pharmacological strategies aiming at activating BAT have encountered limitations due to their lack of specificity and potential neurological and cardiac side effects.

Cell therapy aims to increase energy expenditure and regulate glucose homeostasis by differentiating non-shivering thermogenic cells *in vitro* and transplanting them into patients. The transplanted cells can be reprogrammed from the patient cells for autologous transplantation. While this circumvents the immune rejection, this requires establishment and validation of cell lines for each patient, carrying a prohibitive cost. Alternatively, strategy using allogeneic PSCs-derived cells could be implemented with cells bioengineered to overcome immune detection [63]. Different strategies obtained activate beige adipocytes, including PSCs differentiation, CRISPR bioengineered HUMBLEs and co-culture with capillaries. However, compared to beige adipocytes, brown adipocytes are more efficient [64]. Several brown adipocytes differentiation protocols have been reported. Wang et al. provided an alternative for the transplantation of brown adipocytes by generating organoids which improve cell survival. Other organoid tissues were developed *in vitro* using PSCs, as retina or brain, but in our knowledge, none were developed for BAT. Obtaining organoids from iPSCs is therefore the next step to be developed. This would be an important step toward regenerative medicine and cell therapy against type 1, type 2 diabetes and obesity, as well as other metabolic disorders.

Acknowledgements

The authors acknowledge funding supports from Institut Pasteur de Lille, INSERM and the Agence Nationale pour la Recherche ANR-10-LABX-0046 (AML). We thank Pr. Corbin Antoine (CIRI, ENS de Lyon) for his advice and critical reading of the manuscript.

Author details

Amine Bouchekioua[1,2,3,4], Olivier Pourquié[2,3,4] and Alicia Mayeuf-Louchart[5]*

1 Department of Biology, École Normale Supérieure de Lyon, Lyon, France

2 Department of Pathology, Brigham and Women's Hospital, Boston, MA, USA

3 Department of Genetics, Harvard Medical School, Boston, MA, USA

4 Harvard Stem Cell Institute, Harvard University, Cambridge, MA, USA

5 Univ. Lille, INSERM, CHU Lille, Institut Pasteur de Lille, Lille, France

*Address all correspondence to: alicia.mayeuf-louchart@inserm.fr

IntechOpen

© 2024 The Author(s). Licensee IntechOpen. This chapter is distributed under the terms of the Creative Commons Attribution License (http://creativecommons.org/licenses/by/3.0), which permits unrestricted use, distribution, and reproduction in any medium, provided the original work is properly cited.

References

[1] Ying Z et al. Role of thermogenic adipose tissue in lipid metabolism and atherosclerotic cardiovascular disease: Lessons from studies in mice and humans. Cardiovascular Research. April 2023;**119**(4):905-918. DOI: 10.1093/cvr/cvac131

[2] Chen H-J, Meng T, Gao P-J, Ruan C-C. The role of brown adipose tissue dysfunction in the development of cardiovascular disease. Frontiers in Endocrinology. 2021;**12**:652246

[3] Becher T et al. Brown adipose tissue is associated with cardiometabolic health. Nature Medicine. 2021;**27**:58-65

[4] Christou N, Efthimiou E. Five-year outcomes of laparoscopic adjustable gastric banding and laparoscopic Roux-en-Y gastric bypass in a comprehensive bariatric surgery program in Canada. Canadian Journal of Surgery. Journal canadien de chirurgie. 2009;**52**:E249-E258

[5] Ahima RS. Adipose tissue as an endocrine organ. Obesity (Silver Spring, Md.). 2006;**14**(Suppl 5):242S-249S

[6] Kuryszko J, Sławuta P, Sapikowski G. Secretory function of adipose tissue. Polish Journal of Veterinary Sciences. 2016;**19**:441-446

[7] Bartelt A et al. Brown adipose tissue activity controls triglyceride clearance. Nature Medicine. 2011;**17**:200-205

[8] Stanford KI et al. Brown adipose tissue regulates glucose homeostasis and insulin sensitivity. The Journal of Clinical Investigation. 2013;**123**:215-223

[9] Nedergaard J et al. UCP1: The only protein able to mediate adaptive non-shivering thermogenesis and metabolic inefficiency. Biochimica et Biophysica Acta. 2001;**1504**:82-106

[10] Seale P et al. PRDM16 controls a brown fat/skeletal muscle switch. Nature. 2008;**454**:961-967

[11] Cinti S. Pink adipocytes. Trends in Endocrinology and Metabolism: TEM. 2018;**29**:651-666

[12] Gunawardana SC, Piston DW. Reversal of type 1 diabetes in mice by brown adipose tissue transplant. Diabetes. 2012;**61**:674-682

[13] Gunawardana SC, Piston DW. Insulin-independent reversal of type 1 diabetes in nonobese diabetic mice with brown adipose tissue transplant. American Journal of Physiology-Endocrinology and Metabolism. 2015;**308**:E1043-E1055

[14] Soler-Vázquez MC, Mera P, Zagmutt S, Serra D, Herrero L. New approaches targeting brown adipose tissue transplantation as a therapy in obesity. Biochemical Pharmacology. 2018;**155**:346-355

[15] Kuryłowicz A, Puzianowska-Kuźnicka M. Induction of adipose tissue browning as a strategy to combat obesity. International Journal of Molecular Science. 2020;**21**:6241

[16] Aherne W, Hull D. Brown adipose tissue and heat production in the newborn infant. The Journal of Pathology and Bacteriology. 1966;**91**:223-234

[17] Lean ME. Brown adipose tissue in humans. The Proceedings of the Nutrition Society. 1989;**48**:243-256

[18] Nedergaard J, Bengtsson T, Cannon B. Unexpected evidence

for active brown adipose tissue in adult humans. American Journal of Physiology-Endocrinology and Metabolism. 2007;**293**:E444-E452

[19] Mayeuf-Louchart A et al. Glycogen dynamics drives lipid droplet biogenesis during brown adipocyte differentiation. Cell Reports. 2019;**29**:1410-1418.e6

[20] Ahmed B, Sultana R, Greene MW. Adipose tissue and insulin resistance in obese. Biomedicine & Pharmacotherapy. 2021;**137**:111315

[21] Zelová H, Hošek J. TNF-α signalling and inflammation: Interactions between old acquaintances. Inflammation Research: Official Journal of the European Histamine Research Society. 2013;**62**:641-651

[22] Nieto-Vazquez I et al. Insulin resistance associated to obesity: The link TNF-alpha. Archives of Physiology and Biochemistry. 2008;**114**:183-194

[23] Weir G et al. Substantial metabolic activity of human brown adipose tissue during warm conditions and cold-induced lipolysis of local triglycerides. Cell Metabolism. 2018;**27**:1348-1355.e4

[24] Petrovic N et al. Chronic peroxisome proliferator-activated receptor gamma (PPARgamma) activation of epididymally derived white adipocyte cultures reveals a population of thermogenically competent, UCP1-containing adipocytes molecularly distinct from classic brown adipocytes. The Journal of Biological Chemistry. 2010;**285**:7153-7164

[25] Vegiopoulos A et al. Cyclooxygenase-2 controls energy homeostasis in mice by de novo recruitment of brown adipocytes. Science. 2010;**328**:1158-1161

[26] Ishibashi J, Seale P. Medicine. Beige can be slimming. Science. 2010;**328**:1113-1114

[27] Razzoli M, Emmett MJ, Lazar MA, Bartolomucci A. β-Adrenergic receptors control brown adipose UCP-1 tone and cold response without affecting its circadian rhythmicity. FASEB Journal: Official Publication of the Federation of American Societies for Experimental Biology. 2018;**32**:5640-5646

[28] Harms M, Seale P. Brown and beige fat: Development, function and therapeutic potential. Nature Medicine. 2013;**19**:1252-1263

[29] Rao J et al. Reconstructing human brown fat developmental trajectory in vitro. Developmental Cell. 2023:S1534-5807(23)00397-0

[30] Wang W et al. Ebf2 is a selective marker of brown and beige adipogenic precursor cells. Proceedings of the National Academy of Sciences of the United States of America. 2014;**111**:14466-14471

[31] Rajaii F et al. Temperature and species-dependent regulation of browning in retrobulbar fat. Scientific Reports. 2021;**11**:3094

[32] Miwa H, Era T. Tracing the destiny of mesenchymal stem cells from embryo to adult bone marrow and white adipose tissue via Pdgfrα expression. Development. 2018;**145**:dev155879

[33] Cohen P et al. Ablation of PRDM16 and beige adipose causes metabolic dysfunction and a subcutaneous to visceral fat switch. Cell. 2014;**156**:304-316

[34] Valencak TG, Osterrieder A, Schulz TJ. Sex matters: The effects of

biological sex on adipose tissue biology and energy metabolism. Redox Biology. 2017;**12**:806-813

[35] Auclair M, Roblot N, Capel E, Fève B, Antoine B. Pharmacological modulation of RORα controls fat browning, adaptive thermogenesis, and body weight in mice. American Journal of Physiology-Endocrinology and Metabolism. 2021;**320**:E219-E233

[36] Braz GRF et al. Chronic serotonin reuptake inhibition uncouples brown fat mitochondria and induces beiging/browning process of white fat in overfed rats. Life Sciences. 2020;**245**:117307

[37] Villarroya F, Cereijo R, Villarroya J, Giralt M. Brown adipose tissue as a secretory organ. Nature Reviews Endocrinology. 2017;**13**:26-35

[38] Lau P et al. Rorα deficiency and decreased adiposity are associated with induction of thermogenic gene expression in subcutaneous white adipose and brown adipose tissue. American Journal of Physiology-Endocrinology and Metabolism. 2015;**308**:E159-E171

[39] Monnier C, Auclair M, Le Cam G, Garcia M, Antoine B. The nuclear retinoid-related orphan receptor ROR α controls circadian thermogenic programming in white fat depots. Physiological Reports. 2018;**6**:e13678

[40] Braz GRF et al. Fluoxetine administration in juvenile overfed rats improves hypothalamic mitochondrial respiration and REDOX status and induces mitochondrial biogenesis transcriptional expression. European Journal of Pharmacology. 2020;**881**:173200

[41] Mukherjee J, Baranwal A, Schade KN. Classification of therapeutic and experimental drugs for brown adipose tissue activation: Potential treatment strategies for diabetes and obesity. Current Diabetes Reviews. 2016;**12**:414-428

[42] O'Mara AE et al. Chronic mirabegron treatment increases human brown fat, HDL cholesterol, and insulin sensitivity. The Journal of Clinical Investigation. 2020;**130**:2209-2219

[43] Blondin DP et al. Human brown adipocyte thermogenesis is driven by β2-AR stimulation. Cell Metabolism. 2020;**32**:287-300.e7

[44] Straat ME et al. Stimulation of the beta-2-adrenergic receptor with salbutamol activates human brown adipose tissue. Cell Reports Medicine. 2023;**4**:100942

[45] Wang C-H et al. CRISPR-engineered human brown-like adipocytes prevent diet-induced obesity and ameliorate metabolic syndrome in mice. Science Translational Medicine. 2020;**12**:eaaz8664

[46] Corvera S, Solivan-Rivera J, Yang Loureiro Z. Angiogenesis in adipose tissue and obesity. Angiogenesis. 2022;**25**:439-453

[47] Takahashi K, Yamanaka S. Induction of pluripotent stem cells from mouse embryonic and adult fibroblast cultures by defined factors. Cell. 2006;**126**:663-676

[48] Nishio M et al. Production of functional classical brown adipocytes from human pluripotent stem cells using specific hemopoietin cocktail without gene transfer. Cell Metabolism. 2012;**16**:394-406

[49] Chal J et al. Generation of human muscle fibers and satellite-like cells from

human pluripotent stem cells in vitro. Nature Protocols. 2016;**11**:1833-1850

[50] Liu Y, Fu W, Seese K, Yin A, Yin H. Ectopic brown adipose tissue formation within skeletal muscle after brown adipose progenitor cell transplant augments energy expenditure. The FASEB Journal. 2019;**33**:8822-8835

[51] Konermann S et al. Genome-scale transcriptional activation by an engineered CRISPR-Cas9 complex. Nature. 2015;**517**:583-588

[52] Herzig S, Shaw RJ. AMPK: Guardian of metabolism and mitochondrial homeostasis. Nature Reviews Molecular Cell Biology. 2018;**19**:121-135

[53] Jankovic A et al. Targeting the NO/superoxide ratio in adipose tissue: Relevance to obesity and diabetes management. British Journal of Pharmacology. 2017;**174**:1570-1590

[54] Tran K-V et al. The vascular endothelium of the adipose tissue gives rise to both white and brown fat cells. Cell Metabolism. 2012;**15**:222-229

[55] Min SY et al. Human 'brite/beige' adipocytes develop from capillary networks, and their implantation improves metabolic homeostasis in mice. Nature Medicine. 2016;**22**:312-318

[56] Gealekman O et al. Depot-specific differences and insufficient subcutaneous adipose tissue angiogenesis in human obesity. Circulation. 2011;**123**:186-194

[57] Zhang L et al. Generation of functional brown adipocytes from human pluripotent stem cells via progression through a paraxial mesoderm state. Cell Stem Cell. 2020;**27**:784-797.e11

[58] Su S et al. A renewable source of human beige adipocytes for development of therapies to treat metabolic syndrome. Cell Reports. 2018;**25**:3215-3228.e9

[59] Chal J, Pourquié O. Making muscle: Skeletal myogenesis in vivo and in vitro. Development (Cambridge, England). 2017;**144**:2104-2122

[60] Carobbio S et al. Unraveling the developmental roadmap toward human brown adipose tissue. Stem Cell Reports. 2021;**16**:1010

[61] Wang O et al. Fabricating 3-dimensional human brown adipose microtissues for transplantation studies. Bioactive Materials. 2023;**22**:518-534

[62] Lei Y, Jeong D, Xiao J, Schaffer DV. Developing defined and scalable 3D culture systems for culturing human pluripotent stem cells at high densities. Cellular and Molecular Bioengineering. 2014;**7**:172-183

[63] Lanza R, Russell DW, Nagy A. Engineering universal cells that evade immune detection. Nature Reviews Immunology. 2019;**19**:723-733

[64] Shabalina IG et al. UCP1 in brite/beige adipose tissue mitochondria is functionally thermogenic. Cell Reports. 2013;**5**:1196-1203